Rapid Weight Loss Hypnosis

A Transforming Guide On A New And Easy Way To Burn Fat And Lose Weight Fast Using Powerful Hypnosis Psychology

Self Help for Women Academy

Rapid Weight Loss Hypnosis

Rapid Weight Loss Hypnosis

© Copyright 2021 by Self Help for Women Academy - All rights reserved.

The following Book is reproduced below with the goal of providing information that is as accurate and reliable as possible. Regardless, purchasing this Book can be seen as consent to the fact that both the publisher and the author of this book are in no way experts on the topics discussed within and that any recommendations or suggestions that are made herein are for entertainment purposes only. Professionals should be consulted as needed prior to undertaking any of the action endorsed herein.

This declaration is deemed fair and valid by both the American Bar Association and the Committee of Publishers Association and is legally binding throughout the United States.

Furthermore, the transmission, duplication, or reproduction of any of the following work including specific information will be considered an illegal act irrespective of if it is done electronically or in print. This extends to creating a secondary or tertiary copy of the work or a recorded copy and is only allowed with the express written consent from the Publisher. All additional right reserved.

The information in the following pages is broadly considered a truthful and accurate account of facts and as such, any inattention, use, or misuse of the information in question by the reader will render any resulting actions solely under their purview. There are no scenarios in which the publisher or the original author of this work can be in any fashion deemed liable for any hardship or damages that may befall them after undertaking information described herein.

Additionally, the information in the following pages is intended only for informational purposes and should thus be thought of as universal. As befitting its nature, it is presented without assurance regarding its prolonged validity or interim quality. Trademarks that are mentioned are done without written consent and can in no way be considered an endorsement from the trademark holder.

Rapid Weight Loss Hypnosis

Table of Contents

INTRODUCTION 8

CHAPTER 1: GASTRIC BAND HYPNOTHERAPY—SATISFACTION WITHOUT SURGERY 10

BECOME FIRST ON NATURE'S WAITING LIST 11
BENEFITS OF HYPNOTIC GASTRIC BAND 12
TREATMENT WITH VIRTUAL GASTRIC BAND 12
ADVANTAGES AND DISADVANTAGES OF THE VIRTUAL GASTRIC BAND 13
BENEFITS OF SEVILLE GASTRIC BAND HYPNOSIS 14
4 ADVANTAGES OF SEVILLE GASTRIC BAND HYPNOSIS 14
WHAT IS THE GASTRIC BAND WITH HYPNOSIS? 16
ADVANTAGES OF GASTRIC BAND WITH HYPNOSIS 17
ADVANTAGES OF HYPNOSIS FOR WEIGHT LOSS 19

CHAPTER 2: WHAT IS ADJUSTABLE RING GASTROPLASTY? 22

CHAPTER 3: THE DANGERS OF OBESITY 24

OBESITY IN FRANCE 25
WORLDWIDE OBESITY 25
DIETS 26

CHAPTER 4: VIRTUAL GASTRIC RING UNDER HYPNOSIS 28

HOW DOES ACCOMPANIMENT WORK? 29
THE VIRTUAL GASTRIC RING PLACED UNDER HYPNOSIS: REALITY OR FAKE? .. 31

CHAPTER 5: WHAT IS THE HYPNOTIC VIRTUAL GASTRIC RING? . 32

IS THIS VIRTUAL GASTRIC RING FOR YOU? 33
HOW DO YOU PLACE THE VIRTUAL GASTRIC BAND? 34
HOW DO YOU MAKE IT WORK FOR YOU TOO? 34
Is Your Goal Realistic? *34*
THERAPEUTIC PROGRAM 35

CHAPTER 6: HYPNOSIS (SHORT INTRODUCTION) 38

DEFINITION 38
SUGGESTIONS 39
PROCESS 40
Acceptance or Permission by the Customer *40*
Induction—Deepening of the Hypnotic State or Trance by Various Techniques *41*

Trance Phases *41*
TECHNIQUES 42
THE OBSERVABLE 43
   The Physical *43*
   The psychological *44*
   Selective attention *44*
DISSOCIATION 45
INCREASED RESPONSE TO SUGGESTION 45
SUBJECTIVE INTERPRETATION 45
TRANCE LOGIC 46
RELAXATION 46
TOPICS 46
HYPNOSIS WORKS, BUT NOT AS YOU THINK 47

CHAPTER 7: HYPNOSIS: A NEW APPROACH TO LOSING WEIGHT . 50

COUPLES' OBESITY SURGERY 53
BECOME AN EXPERT PATIENT IN OBESITY SURGERY 54
BARIOACOACH 55

CHAPTER 8: HOW TO REPROGRAM OUR SUBCONSCIOUS 58

HOW CAN THE SUBCONSCIOUS LIMIT US? 58
   Limiting Sources of Negativity *59*
   Focus Images *60*
   Repeating Realistic Statements *61*
   Working on Brain Waves *62*
THE POWER OF HYPNOSIS IN THERAPY 63
CONSCIOUS AND UNCONSCIOUS MENTAL PROCESSES ARE ASSOCIATED ... 64
THE CONSCIOUS AND UNCONSCIOUS ARE DISSOCIATED 64
THE HYPNOTIC TRANCE 65
LEARNING TECHNIQUES OF HOW TO REPROGRAM YOUR SUBCONSCIOUS ... 66

CHAPTER 9: THE MEDITATIVE HYPNOSIS TECHNIQUE IN 5 SIMPLE MOVES 68

THE PREPARATION 69
GET COMFORTABLE AND BREATHE! 70
MEDITATION 71
FIND PEACE 72
ENJOY 72
THE VIEW 73
IDENTIFY THE GOAL 73
GET IT 74
STAY FOCUSED 74
REPETITION 75

CHAPTER 10: HOW TO HYPNOTIZE YOURSELF 78
PREPARING FOR SELF-HYPNOSIS 79
Tuning 81
Project Your Intentions 81
Breathe Deeply 82
Implementation 83
View 84
Emergence 85
THE 3 STAGES OF SELF-HYPNOSIS 85
Step 1: Hypnotic Induction 86
Step 2: Creative Visualization 87
Step 3: Exiting Hypnotic State 87
THE EFFECTS OF AUTO HYPNOSIS ON THE CHEMISTRY OF THE ORGANISM 88
Serotonin 89
Melatonin 90
Endorphins 91
Dehydroepiandrosterone 91
Cortisol 92
Anxiety and Depression 94
Gamma-Aminobutyric Acid 94
Dealing with Premenstrual Syndrome 95
Small But Essential Additional Tips 97
What to Do if I Don't Relax? 98

CONCLUSION 100

Rapid Weight Loss Hypnosis

Introduction

The gastric bandage is a stomach restriction intervention, which is part of the treatments provided by bariatric surgery, also known as pathological obesity surgery.

This can be considered a viable alternative to gastric bypass, vertical gastric resection ("Sleeve"), and biliopancreatic diversion.

Therefore, it is a procedure aimed at limiting food intake and consumption, anticipating the perception of the sense of satiety and consequently promoting weight loss.

The patient will learn to eat less and change their essential eating habits. To undergo this treatment of surgical reduction of stomach volume, you need to contact a specialist.

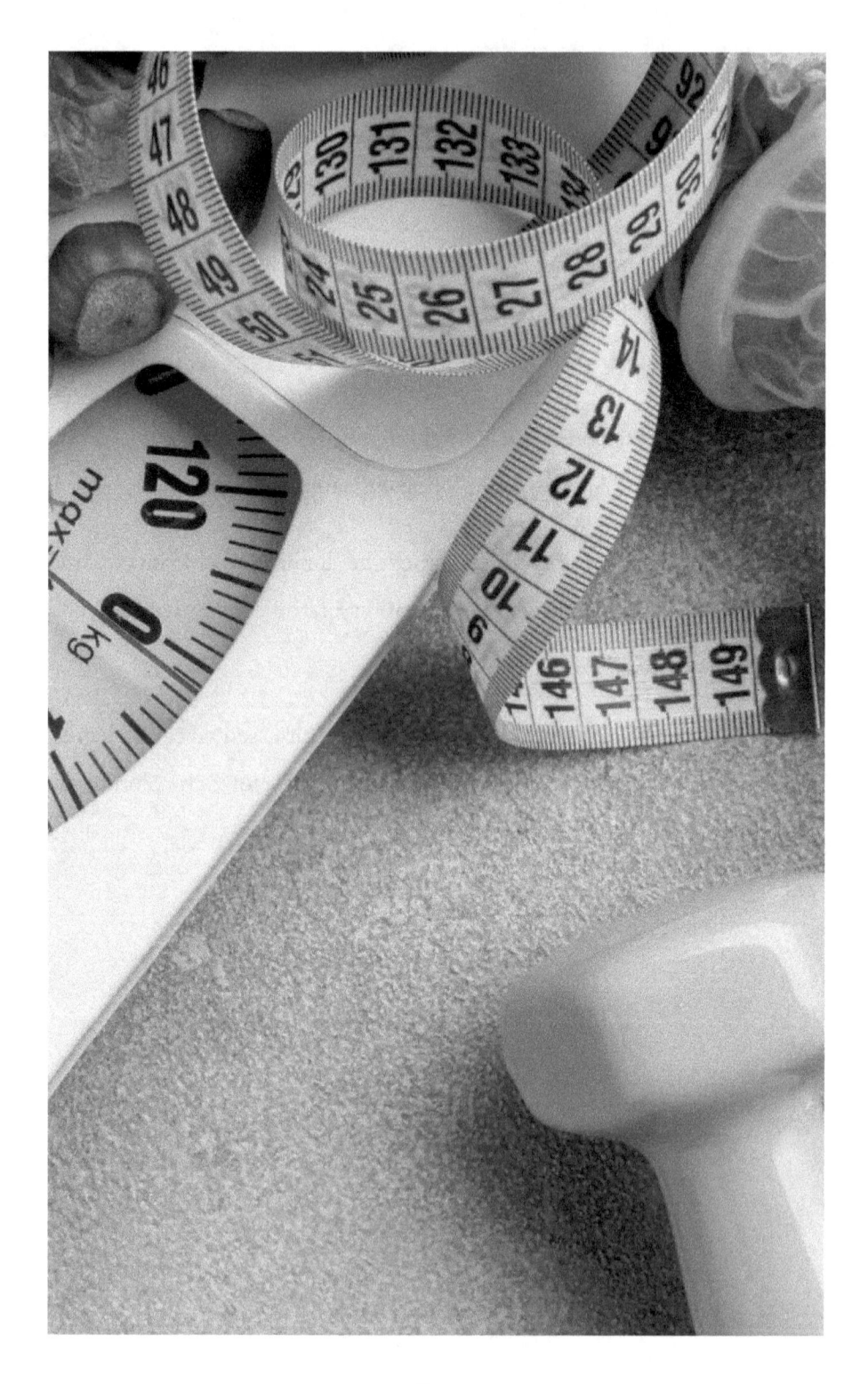

Chapter 1: Gastric Band Hypnotherapy—Satisfaction without Surgery

Putting on a gastric band is a life-saving procedure for many people who have always struggled with their weight, but imagine you can eat like you have a gastric band on without all the stress, cost, and uncertainty of surgery.

With hypnotherapy, it's entirely possible to make your mind believe that there's something physically controlling the size of your portions, even though it's your mental commitment that prevents you from eating more than you would consider healthy.

A hypnotic gastric band can:

- Eliminate or reduce the need for a real gastric band.

- Make the diet much less tedious.

- Help you lose weight quickly but safely.

- Allow you to take full and conscious control of what you put into your body.

Become First on Nature's Waiting List

Not many people are aware of it, but most of the habits you think are immutable are nothing more than reactions in your mind.

Although it might sound like a colossal thing, the brain makes small chemical changes every day in a natural way, so you focus your mind on getting something right.

No habit can't be changed.

Hypnotherapy simply decreases the amount of time it would take you to see a positive change in your life, addressing conflicts subconsciously so you can create the desired changes without having to obsessively correct unwanted behaviors until the brain accepts a new direction.

With gastric band hypnotherapy, the positive impact will not only be clear on your mind and be seen at that slimmer waist.

Unlike having an operation, hypnotherapy has no side effects, which means:

- Do not waste working time.

- No weakness.

- No hospitals or anesthesia.

- No risk.

Benefits of Hypnotic Gastric Band

When everything seemed to stay in diets and weight loss, exercises come to a new technique that, by its application, is nothing like what we are used to seeing in terms of weight loss. The virtual gastric band (BGV) is a method that does not compete with any diet regimen because it is not based on diets or physical activity, but its action is direct on the subconscious.

The virtual gastric band was created by a hypnosis specialist, whose basis his study of obesity globally and the power of mind over people with the disease. Considering that during their research, obese or overweight people went through challenging times throughout their lives, they concluded that stress was directly responsible for the excessive sizes.

Most people reach the goal of losing weight healthily, with proper calorie intake and everyday exercise. However, of this number of people, a reasonably high percentage returns to their previous habits and lost weight. But the main problem is that in some cases, recovery of lost weight is twice as much as what had been eliminated.

Treatment with Virtual Gastric Band

The physical gastric band is performed through surgery. A band is placed in the stomach that closes the stomach bag, cutting it to half its size and causing the person to feel satisfied with little food.

It is an expensive procedure and hard recovery work, both food and mental, because the diet for people with gastric band limits the consumption of certain foods, making the person want them more strongly.

In contrast, the virtual gastric band eliminates virtually all the disadvantages of surgery because it's not surgery even though your brain will think so. It doesn't represent any kind of pain, and you can practice it in sessions by a specialist or get the audio files and listen to them before bedtime.

The treatment works for hypnosis, and you should be in a comfortable and pleasant position. Audio or therapist will make you come into direct contact with your brain until you fall into a restful sleep, and while you sleep, the subconscious thinks you're having surgery with the gastric band, so when you get up, you'll feel it inside.

Advantages and Disadvantages of the Virtual Gastric Band

The most important advantage is that it does not cause any pain in the body. You should lose interest in food from the first session, quickly satisfy yourself with few bites, and not drink liquids during dishes.

The weight will slowly decrease because treatment is not a diet as such. It is a technique that strengthens the brain to avoid overeating and consuming empty calories, which is a disadvantage for those who want to lose weight quickly.

But the virtual gastric band does have a significant disadvantage for people who are up to 25 kilos overweight. In these cases, it is not possible to apply the treatment of the virtual gastric band.

The procedure has a physical therapist cost of about 500 euros, although you can purchase the audio package for less in online stores. However, you must learn to dedicate time to listen to them calmly, as the results may vary by person.

Benefits of Seville Gastric Band Hypnosis

Can real weight be lost through gastric band hypnosis in Seville?

The answer is yes, many of our patients have tried this innovative and efficient method with excellent results, so we will solve all your doubts so that you see the wonders of this method so effective.

4 Advantages of Seville Gastric Band Hypnosis

It is possible to balance the feeling of satiety without having to go through an operating room. Usually, an operation of this type, in addition to having to go through the operating room, its cost ranges between 5,000 and 8,000 euros since, in many cases, Social Security does not accept them.

That's not counting the risks of anesthesia and others added in surgery. We change habits such as continually thinking about food so that we can balance that feeling of satiety.

We help you to know and connect with your body to understand what it needs and, at the right time, not to eat more than necessary.

In short, try to avoid the typical binges that are so bad for diets. It's imperative to know how to stop eating when you're not hungry anymore!

You won't have to worry about the tedious task of counting calories because by applying the new habits acquired, you can eat everything in small amounts.

If you're tired of trying one and a thousand diets that don't work, don't hesitate to try weight loss through hypnosis. You won't regret it. With the gastric band for hypnosis, we teach you how to:

- Free yourself from the diet mentality.

- Change the habits of your diet.

- Listen to your body and learn to take over. You decide what you eat and what you drink at all times.

What Is The Gastric Band With Hypnosis?

It is a method that allows you to lose weight without diets or surgery. The methodology used is hypnosis. I also use other therapeutic modalities such as NLP, coaching, and Gestalt therapy.

It is a process structured in a minimum of 5 sessions, although they may be more oriented to a smooth and utterly personalized hypnosis induction.

The antecedent is found in gastric band surgery by implanting an adjustable silicone ring.

This reduces the volume of the stomach and thus fills it with less food. This creates a feeling of satiety that results in eating less.

This is the secret of the gastric band to lose weight without a diet. The feeling of satiety comes sooner.

However, surgery is intrusive to the body and face, in addition to the risks and discomfort of any surgical intervention.

Hypnosis manages the subconscious so that the body responds as if it had the actual gastric band implanted. In this way, the gastric band with hypnosis replicates the feeling of satiety before it is too late.

You can eat everything but in less quantity, and it's not a forced thing, but simply sense as natural. This is the secret to weight loss without a diet.

Advantages of Gastric Band with Hypnosis

As you can imagine, there are several advantages over surgery with surgery, diets, or weight loss products. Including:

More economical about surgical intervention (in the order of about 6,000 euros and private clinics). Without the risks, discomfort, and postoperative of any intervention. Not everyone can have surgery for health reasons, but they can have the gastric band with hypnosis.

The intervention involves a conscious enjoyment of the food. In this way, you eat less because the feeling of satiety comes sooner. For this reason, you can lose weight without a diet. And not only that, because once the process is finished, you won't have to spend more on select diet products or foods.

Weight loss and weight loss are not the same, but with the gastric band with hypnosis, you can achieve both goals. By convincing the subconscious, through hypnosis that the gastric band has implemented, the feeling of satiety is achieved by ingesting less food. This makes it not necessary to follow any diet or regimen.

Of course, a healthy diet and some additional tips can help, but they are not essential. Optionally, during the process, I provide in writing some additional information and techniques to follow a diet if desired.

Similarly, I consider the previous emotional process, during and after, because I understand that all people are different, and the food mismatches often accompany them with blockages or emotional mismatches. A virtual gastric band with hypnosis and changing habits improves your motivation and self-esteem.

Current neuroscientific advances have confirmed the plasticity of neural connections responsible for habits, so that, once the habit of eating less is implemented, it becomes easier to follow.

Once the habit is already incorporated into the daily routine, you improve your relationship with food and enjoy it more. Also, no more products or additional expenses are needed, and the risks of the yo-yo effect, or rebound effect, are minimized. We are all unique and different beings. For this reason, previous sessions are of great importance because, during them, I take into account all your peculiarities.

Although the gastric band with hypnosis follows a protocol, it is adaptable to each person. The way you deal with difficulties, the way you get motivated, the reasons that induce you to eat, and the eating habits are all these elements. Additional ones I consider to design a unique and personalized induction.

I also record your hypnotic induction in an MP3 file to give it to you. So you can continue to strengthen daily at home for a while. Therefore, it is not a "standard" method, a book, or a manual method. It's a completely personalized process. At your choice, you can follow a few more sessions of emotional support, reinforcement. Also, to follow a specific diet or avoid some foods that you are interested in leaving aside.

Advantages of Hypnosis for Weight Loss

Do you want to lose weight definitively?

Chances are you've already tried different diets or control your diet, but you always get fat again.

You are tired of banning food, of starving

Our weight-loss hypnosis sessions will allow you to change your relationship with food, without anxiety, without prohibitions, and losing weight without starving.

These are the benefits of slimming with hypnosis:

- You will lose weight naturally.

- You will not put on weight again because you will lose weight from the mind and not from the ban.

- You will not go hungry because, with hypnosis, your mind will believe that your stomach is smaller.

- You will change your relationship with food: you will no longer feel that food controls you.

- If you sting between hours, you will no longer have anxiety about eating.

- You will lose weight to your ideal weight quickly and naturally.

Hypnosis is an all-natural technique that will allow you to lose weight without diets and in a healthy way.

With weight-loss hypnosis, you'll acquire new eating habits that you'll lose weight with and never put on weight again.

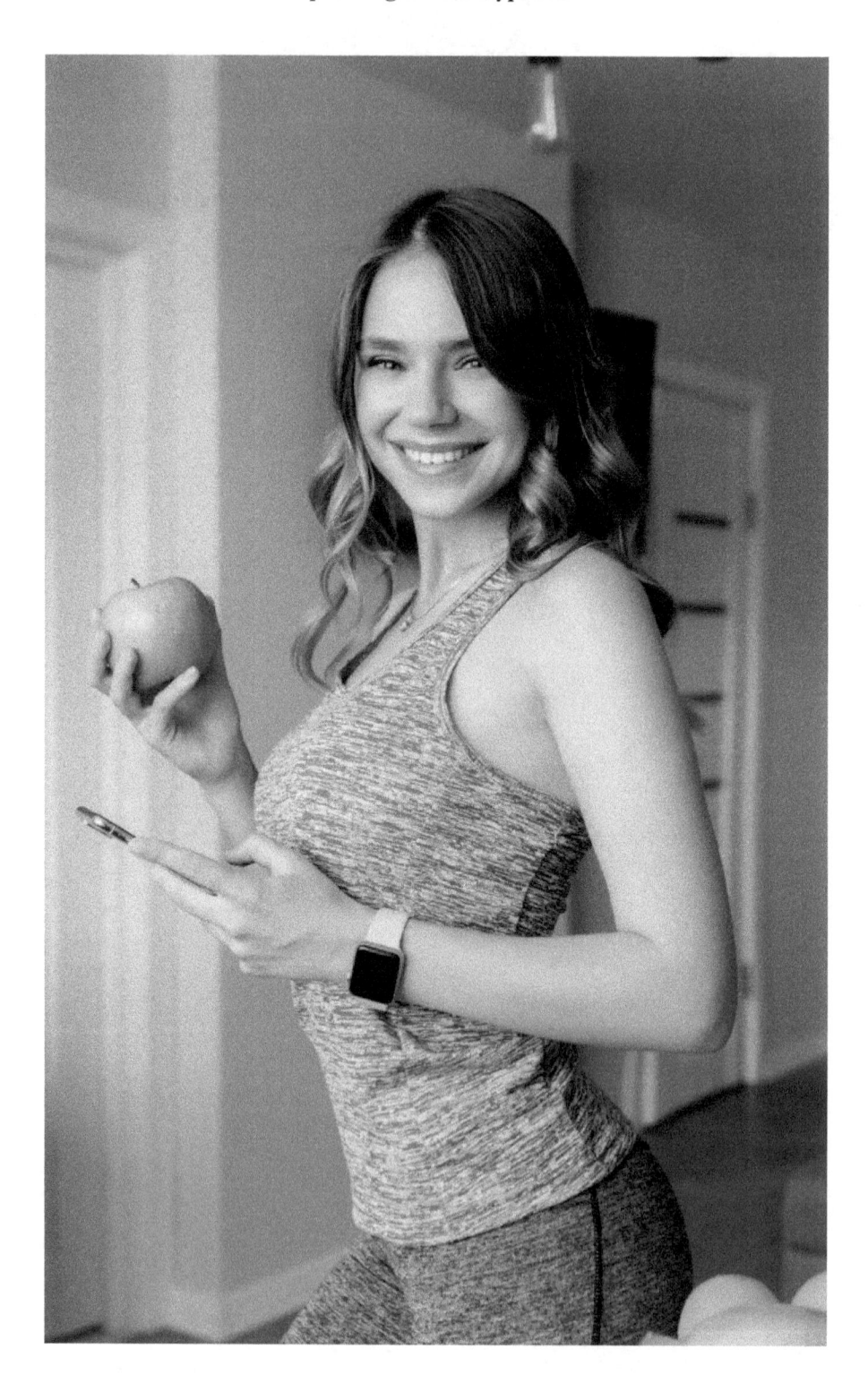

Chapter 2:
What Is Adjustable Ring Gastroplasty?

Gastroplasty is a surgical procedure that involves of permanently placing an adjustable silicone ring around the upper part of the stomach.

This restricts the amount of food a person can absorb.

In France, this operation is covered by social security for people suffering from morbid obesity, i.e., those whose body mass index (BMI) exceeds 40 kg/m2.

Last year, more than 20,000 surgical gastroplasty procedures were performed in France.

Cons of a surgical gastroplasty:

- A very high cost.

- Complications during the operation that even resulted in deaths.

- Hospitalization required.

- Post-operative complications.

- The long healing process.

Only people with morbid obesity can claim to benefit from this operation.

Nausea, reflux, discomfort, and diarrhea are only a small list of side effects experienced after the operation.

Psychological supervision is very often necessary after the operation. Diet, eating habits, and lifestyle are entirely changed and disrupted.

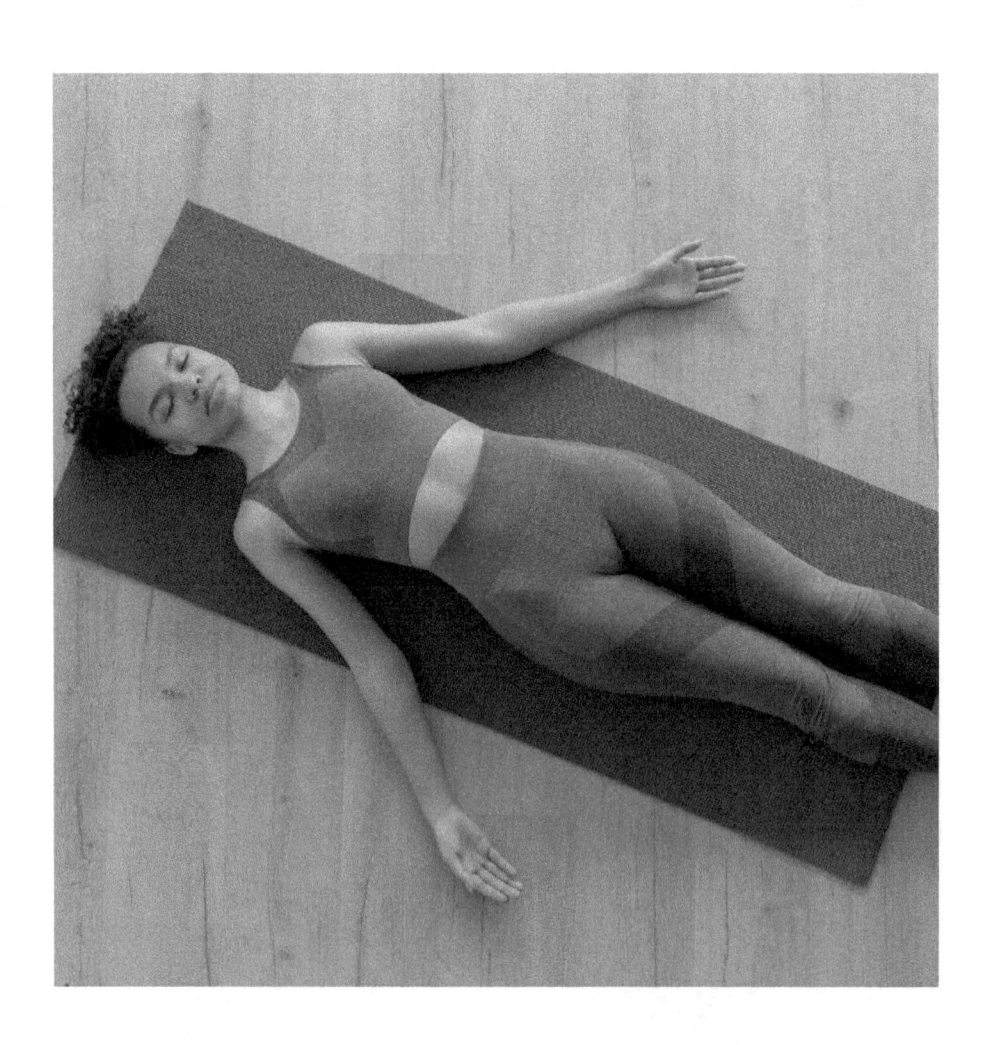

Chapter 3:
The Dangers of Obesity

A serious health risk: It is naïve to think that overweight is only a matter of body image and vanity.

Being obese leads to a low quality of life and can increase the risk of severe and sometimes fatal diseases such as:

- Heart disease.
- Cancer.
- Hypertension.
- Diabetes.

Some of the immediate benefits of weight loss include:

- Less painful joints.
- More energy and flexibility.
- Less shortness of breath during exertion.
- Better self-image.

Obesity in France

While France had one of the lowest obesity rates in Europe, we have been experiencing the same problems as in the United States in recent years. Our increasingly sedentary lifestyle and less healthy month-long diet are at the heart of overweight and obesity. If progress continues at the same rate, one in five people will be obese by 2020.

Obesity, of course, has an impact on health: 55,000 patients die each year from this pathology or one of the disorders associated with obesity.

Moreover, due to the complications of diabetes, obesity is the leading cause of blindness before the age of 65 in France and the leading cause of amputation.

Finally, obesity can become a psychological. Faced with the difficulty of losing their excess weight, some individuals experience great distress that can go as far as depression. Others feel left out or excluded from society.

Worldwide Obesity

Worldwide, 1.5 billion adults over the age of 20 are overweight, and at least 500 million are obese.

According to the World Health Organization, obesity has reached epidemic proportions worldwide. The increase in average weight is observed in all age groups and all socio-economic groups. Even developing countries are not spared.

Diets

Most diets are ineffective at losing weight in the long run. Also, they carry risks such as:

- **Food imbalances:** following a diet often leads to deficiencies.

- **Long-term weight gain:** the caloric restriction imposed by diets is often untenable and generates physical and psychological stress in a state of deprivation, appetite increases, and energy expenditure decreases. The researchers observed that there might be weight loss during the first six months of a diet; however, two to five years later, two-thirds of people regained their lost pounds and even more.

The Hypnotic Gastric Ring provides an alternative for thousands of people undergoing obesity surgery or losing weight sustainably with a diet.

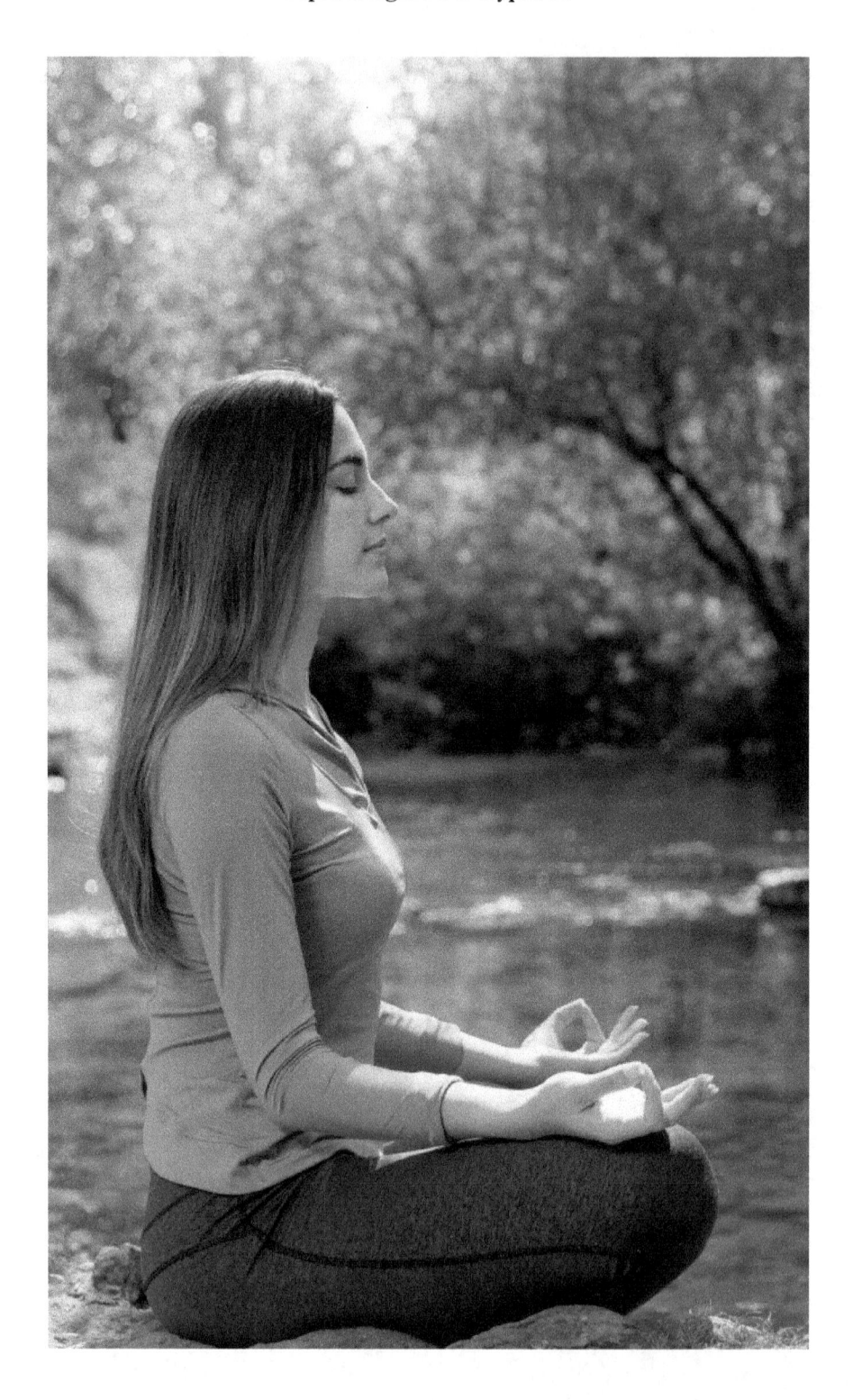

Chapter 4:
Virtual Gastric Ring under Hypnosis

The hypnotic gastric band is for people who have at least 15 to 20kg to lose or a BMI (Body Mass Index) of more than 30.

This is a demanding protocol. In other cases, a classic weight-loss accompaniment by hypnosis will be more suitable.

The gastric band protocol under hypnosis has been developed because being overweight is a real threat to health:

- The risk of death is increased.

- Non-insulin dependent diabetes.

- Cardiovascular diseases.

- Rheumatological problems in the hips, knees, and spine.

- Hormonal abnormalities.

- Venous and skin problems.

- While taking into account the psychological and social impact.

This accompaniment aims to act on the unconscious to alter the feeling of satiety and subconsciously reduce the stomach's size.

It is a question of implanting at the unconscious level the idea and physiological reactions associated with the break of a ring and reprogramming the brain to eat less good and mostly.

The digestion process being completely unconscious, it is possible by hypnosis to deeply anchor a change in eating habits.

Note that the hypnotic gastric band's success rate is more than 80% and higher than that of the surgical gastric band by 67%. But it's not a magic process either.

How fast you lose weight will depend on your determination to follow the protocol.

How Does Accompaniment Work?

This accompaniment will take place in 6 sessions lasting about 1 hour and 30 minutes each, based on a specific protocol. Each session is spaced from 1 week to 1 and a half weeks.

- We will take stock of your situation, your goal.

- We'll highlight the factors that will support your motivation.

- I will give you an information guide on the hypnotic gastric band protocol.

- We'll discuss the golden rules of food.

- You will experience the first contact with hypnosis.

- Tracking developments since the previous session.

- Hypnosis session on feeling full and stopping eating when the stomach is full.

- Tracking developments since the previous session.

- Hypnosis session on stomach contraction.

- Previous sessions have provided preparation. The 4th session is the setting up of the virtual gastric band.

- Following the session, you will need to follow a suitable diet following your stomach's new size.

- Matching the ring to tighten or loosen it depending on how fast you lose weight.

- Weight loss can have significant effects on your life and generate a whole range of changes. This last session aims to accompany you and anticipate these changes so that they do not impact your weight loss.

The Virtual Gastric Ring Placed Under Hypnosis: Reality or Fake?

Faced with the many drawbacks of the gastric band surgically placed, a new method seems to have developed in recent years: installing a virtual gastric band. But what is this virtual gastric band? What is this method? Does it help you lose weight? DocteurBonneBouffe.com conducted its investigation into the pros and cons of this somewhat unusual method.

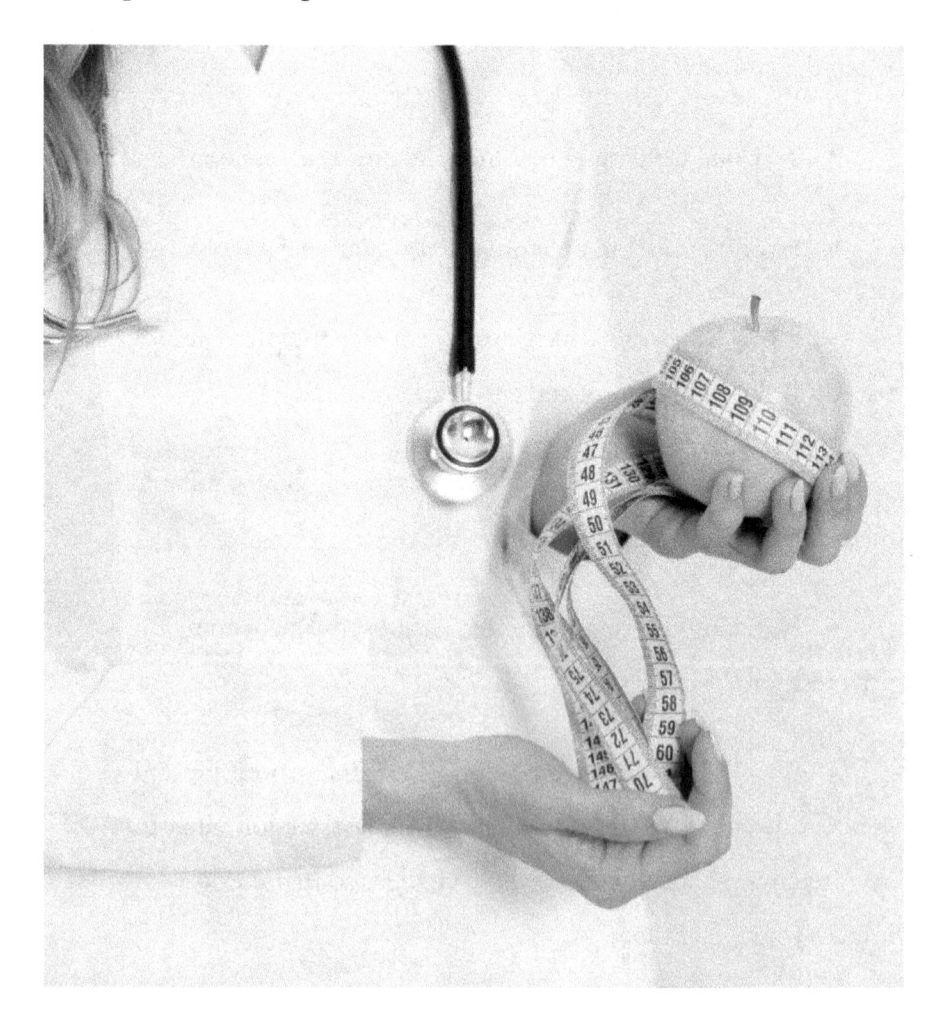

Chapter 5:
What Is the Hypnotic Virtual Gastric Ring?

The gastroplasty, it's like you're experiencing gastric band surgery! You will benefit from the effects similar to the operation but without the inconvenience!

We virtually practice the operation through the HypnoLine method hypnotherapy.

The installation of the virtual gastric band is part of a complete program to lose weight by hypnosis. The big difference is that you don't have to be overweight to be able to access it!

The virtual gastric band under hypnosis will help people suffering from bulimia, snacking, hyperplasia, food compulsion, obsession with diets and calories.

The goal is to break out of the vicious circle of diets, yoyo. Because, as you know, diets are frustrating and weight-gaining.

Thanks to the workshops, I slim down by hypnosis, you will regain the feeling of satiety, and a reduction of appetite is set up naturally.

The workshops are led by Marie-Pierre Preud'homme, hypnosis trainer, hypnotherapist specializing in eating disorders, nutritherapy.

We place a virtual hypnosis ring on the top of the stomach so that it is reduced to a small pocket the size of a golf or tennis ball.

Its volume is adjustable to choose the stomach size that suits you.

- No surgery or post-operative complications!

- Your body and your unconscious ask you for less food, and of course, you meet these new needs.

- The installation of the virtual ring naturally reduces the amount of food.

- You feel full and don't want to eat the extra food you used to eat.

Is This Virtual Gastric Ring for You?

- If you don't want to diet and get frustrated.

- If you do not want surgery, hospitalization of post-operative risks.

- If you want to slim down and maintain your weight over the long term.

How Do You Place the Virtual Gastric Band?

The procedure takes place in 3 sessions:

1. Preparation for the ring placement, setting up the required conditions.

2. Placement of ring.

3. Post-operative management.

We use persuasive techniques!

- Hypnosis view.

- Neuro-linguistic programming.

- Hundreds of people enchanted by the effectiveness of the gastric band!

How Do You Make It Work for You Too?

To make the gastric band as useful for you, check the following:

Is Your Goal Realistic?

For example, if you are 50 years old, aim for weight and silhouette corresponding to your age.

- Are you in a positive frame of mind?

- Do you feel an attitude of welcome and patience?

- Are you ready to invest, to take responsibility?

- You have understood that dysfunctional eating behavior takes time to interfere in your life. It takes time to unlearn it, re-build healthy behavior.

- You're exercising, or you're about to do it.

- Do you know that?

Hypnosis only works if you want to and if you are ready for change, and that's not as obvious as it sounds! You'll find out in the first session. For suggestions to be useful, it is necessary to make them your own. Hypnosis is an active step, a real WORK on oneself!

Therapeutic Program

The program takes place in three sessions. For 21 days, you listen to session 2, preferably always simultaneously, in the same place. Then you listen once a week for four weeks.

Enter NOW in your diary when you decide to do so!

The virtual gastric ring placed under hypnosis:

The gastric band, like any obesity surgery, allows for rapid and massive weight loss. However, it remains a heavy operation with risks. This device could then be replaced by a surprising innovation: the virtual gastric ring. Developed by an English hypnotherapist less than ten years ago, this method is already controversial.

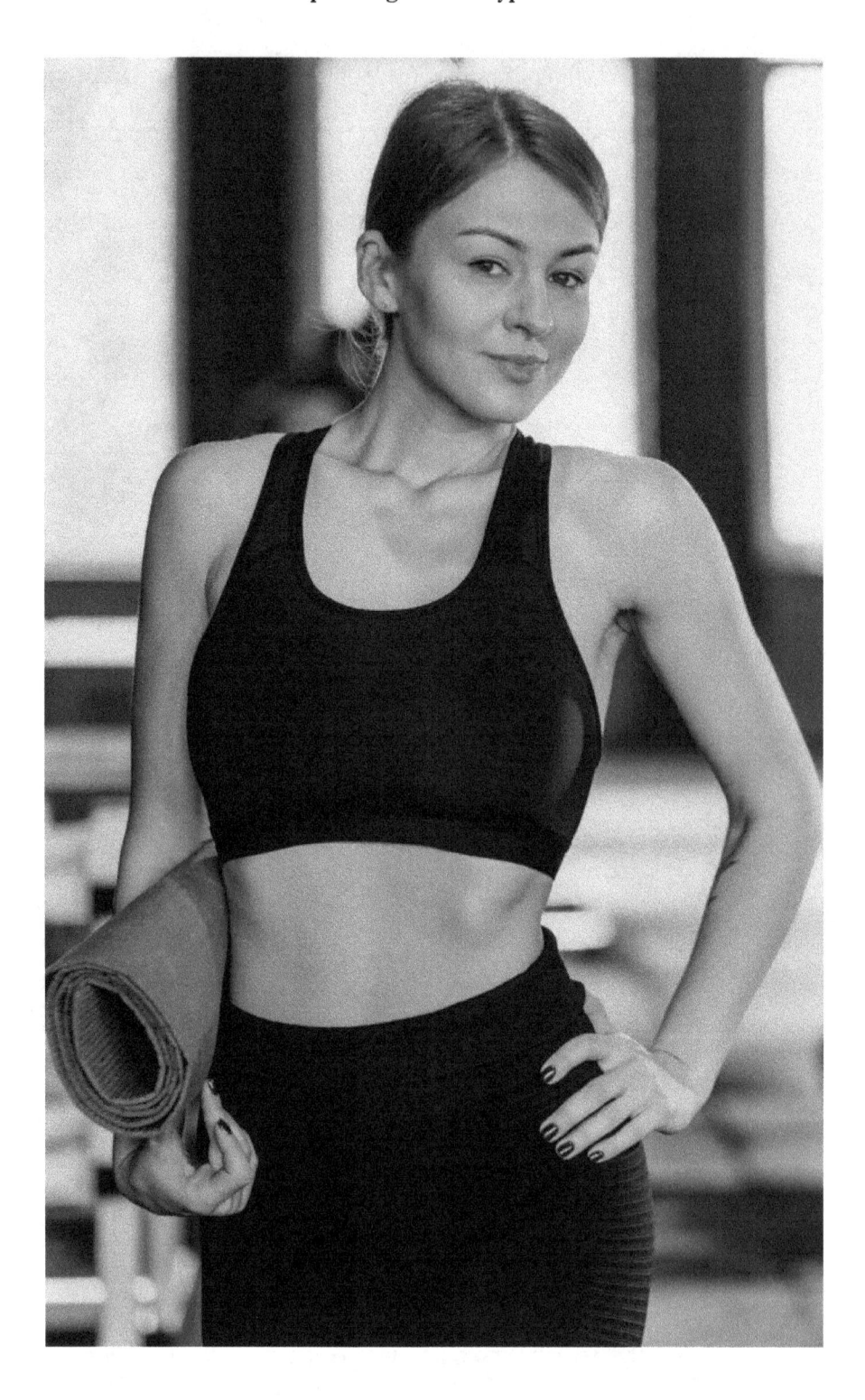

Chapter 6:
Hypnosis (Short Introduction)

Definition

Hypnosis is an altered state of consciousness, self-induced or heater induced, in which both psychological and physiological changes are seen.

This altered state of consciousness, also known as trance or hypnotic state, is located between the conscious and the unconscious, at a midpoint or "unconscious."

This midpoint or unconscious is the Magna route to speak or voluntarily influence, at least try the unconscious.

We assume that the unconscious is where all the information, emotions, and experiences that reach us throughout life are integrated or not integrated into the daily experience.

The unconscious is placed in the non-dominant hemisphere (usually the right), and it is established that its functioning is aortic, timeless, holistic, inductive, symbolic, and integrative.

Away from the criticism, deduction, temporal, and biasing logic of the dominant hemisphere (usually the left).

Suggestions

We are all suggestions able to a greater or lesser extent. It is a characteristic of the species that gives us a particular evolutionary advantage, facilitates and simplifies learning processes.

Suggestions are the material the unconscious will work with. There are nonspecific scripts that can be taken from various books, oriented to different problems.

Non-specification has the advantage that it will be the patient who will attach it to himself even if the therapist is lost. Specificity wants to address the problem directly but can oppress the customer.

Suggestions can be direct, indirect, non-specific, and in the form of fables or metaphors. Its contentment must be positive and acceptable by the client, adapted to their situation and experience; otherwise, it will generate distortion and be rejected or generate a problem of inconsistency and misfit.

Suggestions will make it easier for the customer to see oneself creating forms, overcoming finding alternatives.

Posthypnotic suggestions are intended to facilitate post-trance behaviors. They are based on classic conditioning techniques. Suggestions can alter both physical perception and analgesia and anesthesia, such as psychological perception, affecting self-esteem and willingness to act.

Hypnosis gives suggestions that pretend to be beneficial to the client, but that's the last hypnosis step. The laws of suggestibility were established by Coué (8) and are as follows:

- **Concentrated care act:** The law of focused care means that when a person focuses their attention on an idea, that idea tends to be realized.

- **Law of reversed effort:** This means that when a person thinks they can't do something and then tries, the more they try, the less they try, the less they can do it.

- **Law of dominant affection:** This means that a suggestion linked to emotion will predominate over any other direction found in the mind at that time. Dominant taste (feeling), together with a guide, makes it exert a more significant influence on the mind.

Process

Three points are recognized in a hypnotic process:

Acceptance or Permission by the Customer

Acceptance in one way or another is occurring when the customer comes to the query demanding help. The level of acceptance has to do with the quality of the rapport established in the therapeutic relationship. If it is good, if empathy is felt, approval will be more significant.

This first point is the fundamental premise that must be given to the delay of the following (exception made in the negative trances).

Induction—Deepening of the Hypnotic State or Trance by Various Techniques

Suggestions there is a negative trance, caused for example, by accident in which acceptance is not necessary.

Trance Phases

Hypnotic trance can be considered a naturally produced phenomenon in a continuum of emotional intensity (8). There are four discernible phases in a person's emotional state and three phases of hypnosis:

- **Normal, no hypnosis:** A slight modification of normal behavior.

- **The first phase of hypnosis:** Mass psychology or crowds. Increased suggestibility and tendency to imitation. More changes.

- **The second phase of hypnosis:** Profound muscle inhibition, analgesia, hallucination, "sleepwalking." Extreme changes.

- **The third phase of hypnosis:** Stupor, "suspended animation," anesthesia.

- **In clinical practice:** Positive formal trance is used. Hypnosis can occur less traditionally, whether in a movie, a news story, an ad, or only in a meaningful conversation. We have all experienced some of these trance types, for example, when driving and reaching the destination without knowing how our unconscious is leading us. Having the feeling that five minutes have passed when an hour has passed, our unconscious stops our clock when we are in short; time seems to stop and lengthen otherwise.

Techniques

- **Techniques for induction:** By using the fixation of the look at a point on the wall, or hand in hand and in light. To move on to one's sensations, and relaxation. The tone and cadence of the voice must be different from those of a normal conversation, as we address the unconscious.

- **Techniques for deepening:** Through metaphors or visualizations such as the body of a hot candle, or the eye of the mind, the thousand details of the garden, the mountain road, the spiral staircase. Deepening techniques, such as levitation of the arm during trance, make no sense but an external indicator for the therapist that magic is occurring.

The Observable

The Physical

In the positive trance acts the parasympathetic, opposite, or complementary S.N. of the sympathetic. It deals with the function of restoring functions and storing the necessary resources in difficult situations. The following physiological changes are expected (8, 9):

- Muscle Relaxation.

- With eyes closed, flickering, and eye movements fast.

- Changes in breathing rate and pulse.

- Relaxation of the lower jaw.

- Catalepsy or Inhibition of voluntary movements. Forget the body.

- Increased tear and salivary secretion.

- Decreases heart rate.

- Vascular dilation, particularly in the visceral area.

- Pupil contraction.

- Stimulation of digestive activity.

- Increased of the tone of the bronchial muscles.

- Increased tone and movements of the urinary tract.

- The increased amount of glycogen is deposited in the liver and muscles.

- The tendency to reduce the number of white blood cells with increased eosinophils and lymphocytes.

- The tendency to alkalosis (+).

- Some increase in insulin secretions, parathyroid, and thymus glands.

Changes 1 through 5 are the most easily observable to the naked eye.

The psychological

Psychological characteristics of the hypnotic state, (taken from 9).

Selective attention

It is the ability to deliberately focus on the experience while "disconnecting" from the rest.

Dissociation

The conscious mind deals with hypnotic procedures, while the unconscious actively seeks symbolic meanings, past associations, and appropriate responses.

The fact that conscious and unconscious minds can be divided to some extent and used as independent entities even if they are dependent on is the cornerstone of hypnosis.

Increased Response to Suggestion

The attentional and dissociative factors described above usually lead to an increased response to suggestions.

Increasing the ability to respond to requests is a choice made by the customer and must be guided by someone he/she trusts who can help.

Subjective Interpretation

A person will respond to a word or phrase that is unpredictable. Discover which communications facilitate the hypnotic experience and hinder it are two of the most valuable aspects of training in clinical hypnotherapy with small groups.

Trance Logic

This refers to the customer's need to have a realistic or rational experience.

Relaxation

A person can be hypnotized without necessarily being relaxed, but the relaxation of body and mind is a feature that most people associate with hypnosis.

Peace makes customers feel good, alters their experience of themselves in a well-defined way, and can be convinced, even that they are hypnotized.

Topics

Some topics make the trance experience difficult. Issues that come from the world of the spectacle and the fear of the unknown. It may be worth trying to disarm them:

- You can hypnotize me even if I don't want to: It can't be. No one can be hypnotized against the will; that would go against the first principle necessary for the trance to occur, which coo has been said is acceptance, a salve made from traumatic situations in which the will is violated (accidents, war situations, etc.)

- If I let myself be hypnotized, they can make me do what I do not want to do: In the trance, the consciousness and the will are perfectly preserved so that when a person was asked to do something contrary to the will or ethics, that person does not do it.

- What if I fall asleep and don't wake up, or the psychologist dies of an attack and stays in a trance? From the magic, you can leave in a way suggested by the hypnologist or nature of your own free will when you disagree with what is happening.

- Will I lose control of myself? This fear of being in someone else's hands is perhaps the most common. When the client gets carried away and follows the suggestions they give him, he is the one who gets carried out, and he is the one who follows the transgressions; if I wanted not to, I wouldn't. We see this when we say, "Now you go down step 9 to 8 to 7 to 5," and then he tells us. "Be more careful than if I don't get caught; I kill me, you've made me skip the step 6." He has grabbed himself and had the control to solve the problem, and if he fled, he would have been unsolvable. He would have come out of the trance, not partially as he did, but thoroughly.

Hypnosis Works, but Not as You Think

Hypnosis is a set of techniques surrounded by myths and unfounded mystery. But in reality, its foundation is entirely scientific and is based on the functioning of our brain. Criticized by many, misunderstood by almost everyone, revered by some, and understood by a few, so is hypnosis. The myths amalgamate around it, giving it a pedigree of mystery very appropriate for these dates. What's behind it? Wasn't it a pseudoscience? If it works, can you do whatever you want with it? And if so, why isn't it used more often? Today we tell you what scientists know about it.

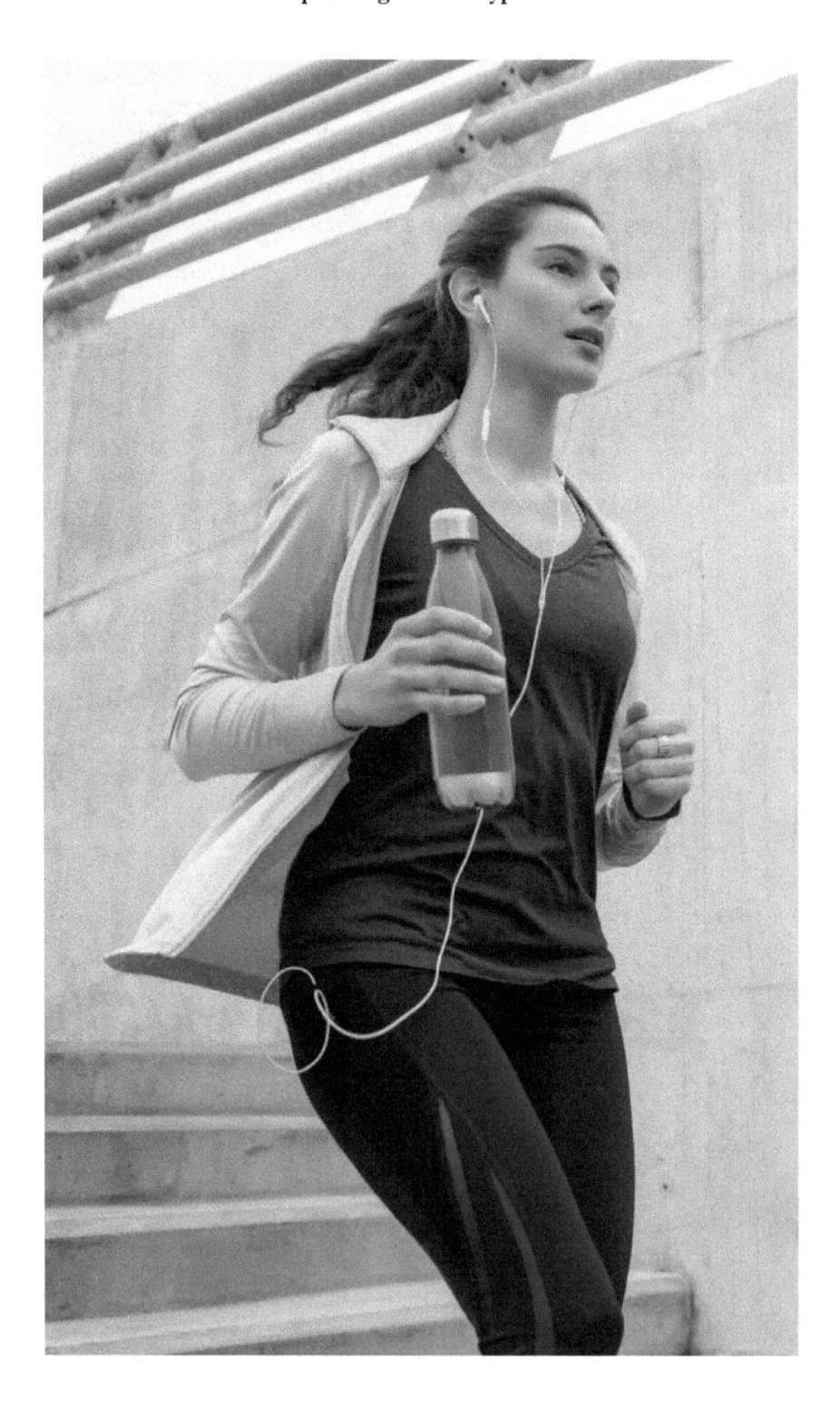

Chapter 7:
Hypnosis: A New Approach to Losing Weight

While diets are known to be ineffective in the long term, obesity surgeries remain massive operations with significant risks. However, this type of process is among the most effective in losing weight quickly and not regaining it.

In 2011, Sheila Granger, a London hypnotherapist, came up with the idea of developing a surprising device: the virtual gastric band. During a hypnosis session, the therapist performs an imaginary operation by placing a gastric band imagined by the patient. Weight loss is real.

Before reaching this critical moment, the practitioner asks the patient about his weight, his difficulties in losing weight, his specific problems concerning food, his goal of weight loss. Once "posed," the virtual gastric band will help to avoid cracking and cause you to lose weight.

Like real bariatric surgery operations, though, the imaginary gastric ring is just a tool. No magic here. If you don't get involved in the process, it doesn't work. It should also be noted that several hypnosis sessions are necessary to carry out this process. This requires an investment of time but also money.

A virtual gastric band that is already not unanimous.

Although very recent, this weight-loss method does not please everyone. It must be said that unlike very real obesity surgeries, it is not strictly regulated by law. You don't have to have a BMI that puts us in moderate, severe, or morbid obesity to benefit from it. A Top Santé journalist had an imaginary gastric band put down to go from a size 38 to 36, she says.

Even more surprising, some sites market recordings of self-hypnosis to be able to carry out this imaginary operation yourself. What happens then when this method lands in the hands of a person suffering from eating disorders? Again, the lack of framing and rules around the virtual gastric band raises questions.

In 2016, the authorities warned against hypnosis-absorbing therapies. At issue is some very poorly trained professionals who start practicing. Marie Arnaud, a hypnotherapist for 30 years, told the newspaper 20 minutes:

"I met a patient who had started terrible diarrhea to lose weight thanks to a self-hypnosis protocol available on the internet. She ended up in the hospital."

Suppose the virtual gastric band can give a boost to those who are starting a weight loss process. In that case, it is, therefore, advisable to turn to a qualified professional, having received training at the French Institute of Hypnosis (IFH) or the French Confederation of Hypnosis and Brief Therapies (CFHTB).

As always, the more enticing the promises, the more caution is required. And you, have you ever tested hypnosis to lose weight? What do you think of this gastric band? We talk about it on the forum.

Stéphane Tomasso underwent a sleeve surgery in 2015. Thanks to this bariatric surgery, he lost 63 kilos. It changed his life and that of his couple. What to do with this experience? He's telling us his story.

The day Stéphane decided to have surgery on a sleeve.

Stéphane Tomasso was a happy man. Big, but comfortable. His entourage was worried about his obesity, but after trying all the diets, he didn't want to hear about his weight anymore. Obesity surgery was not for him either. He was married, fulfilled in his work as a specialized educator. Everything was fine.

And then one day, a kind of click. His wife, herself obese, decides to start a course of obesity surgery. She eventually persuaded Stéphane to follow her to one of the patient meetings. He decided to embark on the adventure as well. He weighs 153 kilos, and his Body Mass Index is 51.

A fulfilling professional career, but which also gave way to glossophobia.

At this time, Stéphane is also pleased professionally. After starting his career as a neighborhood leader in 1995, he graduated as a specialized educator in 2009. He then worked in contact with people with autism or addictology.

Obesity is not a problem. He is invested and appreciated by his hierarchy and the people he supports. A physique is finally reassuring for the public and those in charge of structures who see him as a great fellow who can intervene in the event of a violent situation.

Despite everything, he remains hurt by a few remarks, such as that of a journalist coming to interview him on his profession and who will describe him as a "chubby mocking." Stigmatizing words such as all overweight people can receive. Stories that leave traces, which pushed him all his life to diet after diet and gained more weight.

Couples' Obesity Surgery

Therefore, as a couple Stéphane Tomasso and his wife embark on "the adventure of bariatric surgery." He had sleeve surgery in July 2015, and his wife had a bypass the following month.

While we now know that bariatric surgery often involves risks concerning stability in couples, precisely the opposite will happen here: "I can say that this operation has further strengthened our relationship: we knew how to support each other, and each understood what the other was going through.

On a personal level, this operation not only changed our lives but made it more beautiful: we travel without fear of the eyes of others, enjoy life to the fullest, and are more accomplices than ever."

In total, he will lose 63 kilos and his wife 65 kilos thanks to the bariatric surgery.

Become an Expert Patient in Obesity Surgery

During his course of obesity surgery, Stéphane Tomasso decided to create a Facebook page, "La Sleeve de Stéphane," to share his experience. A real success and a source of experience sharing, which now has 3,400 fans.

The story could have ended there, but Stéphane is curious, an enthusiast who asks himself many questions about what happens beyond the surgery.

He quickly understands that to put all the chances of success on his side, the sleeve or bypass is not limited to an intervention but requires real support.

In 2018, he resumed his studies to obtain a university diploma in therapeutic education for the patient.

With his experience as a specialized educator, he has worked a lot on emotional deprivation, whether with children in foster care or recently with people in a situation of addiction.

The link between all this seemed evident to him: emotional eating (we eat to fill a void or to face a negative emotion): "There is often a correlation between" abnormal, "weight gain and psycho-trauma."

Barioacoach

Personalized support for patients wishing to benefit from a sleeve or a bypass. Stephane then decided to create Bariacoach.com in January 2018. His project: to offer personalized support to work on comprehensive care for patients choosing to have obesity surgery.

Aware that he could not alone hold all the keys allowing each person to find the resources they needed, he then created a network of professionals.

Barioacoach now has no less than 23 people, all specialized, trained, and informed in the specific nature of the care of people wishing to benefit from a sleeve or a bypass or who have already been operated on 13 dieticians, four sophrologists, one clinical psychologist, two sports coaches trained in Adapted Physical Activity (APA), one yoga teacher, one hypnosis master practitioner, and himself (patient-expert in obesity and project coordinator).

Very committed, Stéphane Tomasso wants to go even further by developing therapeutic workshops (cooking, self-esteem, well-being, sport, and health, etc.), the organization of conferences with authors who have written on the subject or with associations such as Stop TCA (Food Behavior Disorders).

With Bariacoach.com, he also wants to set up training actions for social medico professionals (training centers for specialized educators, social workers, etc.) and work with local communities to fight glossophobia.

Interestingly, this course is to note that beyond the technical gesture of obesity surgery, it is all that there is around that allows to guard against failure, regaining weight, and can also be the depression, which results and can sometimes lead to alcoholism and suicide.

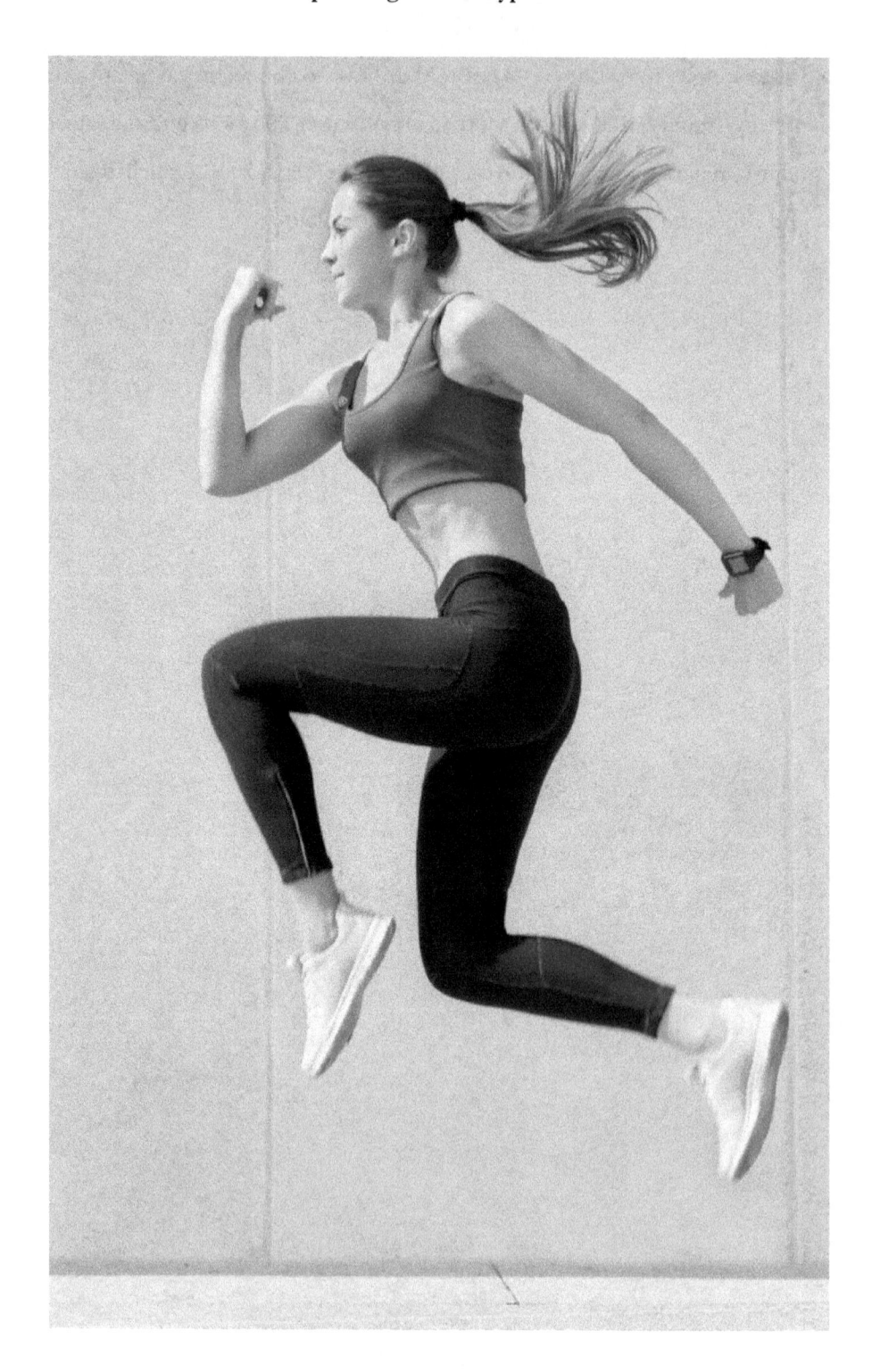

Chapter 8:
How to Reprogram Our Subconscious

We now know that our subconscious has immense power over the control of our life experiences. It also has some on our success.

The subconscious helps us choose our food to interact with others, reality, stress.

It also directly affects our success by stimulating or not our will and ambitions.

If you find yourself in trouble to carry out your professional projects, you may have just met your subconscious for the first time despite your repeated efforts.

Here's why and especially how to reprogram it; so it doesn't fail to succeed.

How Can The Subconscious Limit Us?

We become aware of our subconscious only when we discover its negative power over our life. The rest of the time, we live with it without paying attention. It is like the backstage of our consciousness. It brings together our intuitions, our fears, our experiences, our beliefs (including limiting).

The subconscious appears to us only when we find ourselves in the grip of a desire for success that we fail to realize, without objective reasons. This existing perception began to form from the beginning of our lives, but initially, it was done without differentiation between reality and our inner self before our consciousness was formed.

In general, having a subconscious is useful since it feeds the conscious level through emotions, intuitions, and personal experiences. This becomes problematic when it limits our progress, especially concerning a balanced, successful, or prosperous life.

Apart from any pathological character, we can lift our limiting beliefs and reprogram our subconscious ourselves gradually. We can do this in two ways concerning our professional success.

Limiting Sources of Negativity

We live in a very comfortable society in more ways than one but where anxiety syndromes have increased considerably:

- Fear of missing out linked to inflationary consumption needs;

- Fear of the other connected to a civilization that has become over-urbanized, losing ancestral social and solidarity ties.

- Fear of the future, related to constant over-information, which leaves little critical recoil.

Freeing oneself from some of this negativity allows finding space in your head to receive more positive messages that will enable us to regain specific mental hygiene and peace of heart without falling into the inverse excess of an unrolled optimism.

Focus Images

Visualization is a great way to reprogram one's mind with lively and stimulating images.

We are spending even 10 to 15 minutes a day visualizing festive scenes of our lives changes everything. Watching something we love helps calm the heartbeat, soothes our mind, and regains our intuitions' particular fluidity.

Daily and regular practice leads to a lasting reprogramming of negative experiences.

Meditation, relaxation, yoga, and sophrology allows contact with the breath. Only create a breathing and oxygenation space at the heart level, resulting in more constructive mental effects and images.

This gradually reconditions our subconscious with reassuring, soothing, positive, and meaningful emotions and images for us.

Repeating Realistic Statements

Of course, there is the Coué method in this council, but with a precaution to take: not to affirm things that one does not believe in, such as "I am very successful!"

Instead, I prefer realistic statements such as "I like the idea that I can succeed, and I give myself complete resources. I act accordingly every day."

The idea is to focus on a present, not future, condition. Our subconscious, mostly when it is failing, reacts badly to the future because it imposes additional pressure on a current evil being.

Living and acting in the present, on the other hand, is very useful because it restores the power of immediate action, even and above all, from small things.

Moreover, our subconscious is not 'blind': repeating 'I am good,' while the reality is the opposite, has a counterproductive effect, sending it contradictory messages. Base your statements solely on emotions you feel: "I am good when I think I have every means in me to succeed by acting step by step, constructively."

It doesn't take more than that to lift mountains!

Statements don't work if you just say them from time to time. Recite them often, three times in a row, and slowly.

Working on Brain Waves

Today you find a plethora of music, sounds, and audios to free yourself from tension, think positively, and meditate in an accompanied way in music or by voice.

It's no coincidence! Sounds change the frequency of brain waves.

Your brain waves fall into a specific frequency depending on what you do at a given time:

- Gamma when you are engaged in certain motor functions;

- Beta when you are fully conscious and actively focused;

- Alpha when you're relaxed;

- Theta when you are tired or a little sleepy;

- Delta when you sleep soundly.

Research has shown that your subconscious is more receptive to positive reprogramming when one is relaxed and related to alpha or theta states.

Our subconscious then drops its defenses and can absorb the message we want to program.

It is a phenomenon that occurs during meditations, hypnosis, or self-hypnosis, for example.

The Power of Hypnosis in Therapy

I wrote about "What is coaching," I commented that I would talk about hypnosis as a tool for change. I want to explain to you what the power of hypnosis is in therapy.

We are used to associating the word hypnosis with sometimes esoteric or magical concepts, which leads us to have a skeptical attitude. Hypnosis is indeed a discipline used to make magic shows, in which the hypnotist has complete power over the hypnotized person. In that case, however, hypnosis is a handy and useful tool in therapy.

The two types of hypnosis, theatrical and therapeutic. They differ from each other by the purpose for which it is practiced.

- **Theatrical hypnosis:** It's a form of spectacle, entertainment for the public.

- **Therapeutic hypnosis:** It's a form of therapy. The power of hypnosis in medicine is unquestionable.

Both also have one thing in common: under no circumstances does the hypnotist or therapist have any power or control over the will of the hypnotized person, who is conscious at all times.

In Today's article, I would like to talk to you about what one of them is and how one of them works, therapeutic hypnosis, the power of hypnosis in therapy, and how it can help many people solve problems that they cannot do consciously and rationally.

When I started forming at Ericksonian Hypnosis, my teacher, Teresa García, of the Milton Erickson Institute in Madrid, explained what I now want to share with you. We all know that several states or levels of sleep are associated with specific brain activity (deep sleep, REM, etc.) Similarly, there are several stages of wakefulness, mainly two: conscious and unconscious mental processes are associated and one in which they dissociate. What does this mean?

Conscious and Unconscious Mental Processes Are Associated

It represents the most common wakefulness, which accompanies us during most of the day's activities. In this state, our conscious attention creates a right filter through which any order, advice, idea, or suggestion are carefully analyzed through the magnifying glass of rationality. It's like we have an activated continuous defense mechanism. In this way, everything they tell us, for the sake of coming to us, crashes into this wall, and our beliefs, fears, values manipulate the information.

The Conscious and Unconscious Are Dissociated

It is characterized by a dissociation between our conscious and unconscious parts. This state is what we call hypnotic trance, and our conscious attention is focused on one point. Doing so creates a space, a passage through which every message can directly reach our unconscious, without manipulation or filters. During the hypnotic trance, the person enters a state of intense relaxation. He hears the therapist's voice and the messages (metaphors, stories, suggestions, anecdotes) that he uses to guide his unconscious towards the resources he needs to solve his problem.

The Hypnotic Trance

Hypnotic trance is nothing more than a natural state of our mind, and we all experience it, unknowingly, many times throughout the day. I'll give you an example: Have you ever had to drive your car, get to your destination, and suddenly realize that you haven't been aware of it? It's like you've launched an autopilot when it comes to driving. In doing so, your mind has dissociated from the practical act of driving and connected with your inner world, your emotions, and ideas. If it happened to you, you've experienced a hypnotic trance, too.

The most recent research has revealed that when we are hypnotized, something exciting happens at the neural level: Our mind cannot distinguish whether what it "visualizes" during hypnosis is real or not. Here's another simple example:

If during hypnosis, I am visualizing myself walking, the same neurons will activate if I were roaming. If I imagine myself walking in a normal state (not under hypnosis), other neurons are activated, those related to imagination and creativity. That is, during the hypnotic trance, the mind comes to live an experience. This discovery explains to us even more clearly why hypnosis can help re-framing past events and building personal resources for the present and the future.

Learning Techniques of How to Reprogram Your Subconscious

Were you interested in knowing more about the subconscious? We know you do, and you're in the right place.

We know that the mind is a complex organ of the human body. It is surprising to learn about the mind's functioning when a person is fully conscious and in a subconscious state. However, you may have wanted to change yourself and your thoughts to be a new person many times.

Before you can be a new person, you need to think about who you want to be and visualize it.

Here are some ways you can learn techniques for renewing or reprogramming your subconscious mind.

The first thing is that positive statements have to be made. You have to boost your mind with positive and satisfying questions and answers. For example, make statements like, "I'm pleased I've done my job." This is a positive statement and works excellent for subconscious minds.

Visualization is an important property that helps you become a new man and plays an essential role in your subconscious mind's power. This visualization should be creative, and you must have the ability to think and feel the things you want in life. It means you must be able to imagine it with your eyes closed. The display property plays an essential role in the subconscious mind.

Audios are also a way to push the subconscious mind to a higher level. Here you reach a high concentration. For example, if you hear some positive words silently at night on an audio player, even while you're asleep, it impacts your mind and plays the affirmation role in the subconscious mind. Take the test, and you'll be surprised!

However, there are also many other ways to increase the power of your mind. Processes like hypnosis, EFT, and sublime videos also make an impact on your subconscious mind. The steps to program your subconscious mind once again are simple but, for some, challenging to follow.

Words and emotions influence the subconscious mind more than elsewhere. This is why you have the power to attract more things when you are in a state of happiness because, at that moment, the subconscious mind is full of affirmations and visualizations.

Therefore, the mind is a very complicated process that you must spend years and understand its pattern of functioning through study if you want to study. You can follow the tips we gave you and perform these exercises. You will start to notice the change immediately.

Chapter 9:
The Meditative Hypnosis Technique in 5 Simple Moves

Now you are ready to be introduced to the technique that will allow you to connect with your subconscious. As you'll find out shortly, you'll notice that the method itself is straightforward, but it doesn't have to be simplified.

That is, do not doubt its effectiveness because its power lies in the fact that you first have to believe it, and above all, it will take time to see the first results.

Constant practice, as for meditation, is the key to the success and effectiveness of the technique.

The four actions that characterize the self-hypnosis technique are:

- The preparation.
- Meditation.
- The view.
- Repetition.

Below you will find all the insights for each point. Are you ready?

Well, let's get started!

The Preparation

Experience shows that if you predict from afar the design you want to undertake, you can quickly act once it comes to execute it.

As in everything, good preparation will make it easier for you to succeed in what you want to achieve.

Comfortable clothes and a full belly the first thing you will have to do for good preparation is to wear comfortable clothes. Prefer clothing that won't make you feel cold. A warm temperature will help our body relax more, and you will feel enveloped by a comfortable feeling.

It is also recommended not to prepare on an empty stomach, as you may be easily distracted by hunger bites. Even an overly substantial meal could get in your way. So I recommend you have a light meal a couple of hours before you start. You must have the right energy for intense meditation and concentration activity. If you are too satiated, you risk quickly falling into the temptation of sleep.

Find a quiet place and eliminate distractions.

The preparation is very similar, if not the same as meditation, as it is what you will do. Although with some small changes!

Then head to your safe place, where you can rest comfortably and where you won't be interrupted or disturbed. It can be your room or any room in the house. If you're on the go, or if you get the chance where you live, you might prefer to be in touch with nature. Maybe in the mountains, at sea, in the garden, it doesn't matter. The important thing is that it is a place that transmits you peace and security, where you know you can rest easy!

For added security, be sure to eliminate any source of external interference and distraction. Turn off your cell phone. These minutes you will have to dedicate them entirely to yourself. If you are perhaps at home or with friends, kindly ask to leave your privacy and not disturb yourself for the time necessary for this practice.

Get Comfortable and Breathe!

Well, now you're ready to start. So take a convenient position, which you know won't bother you for 15 or 30 minutes. The time of the exercise depends solely on you. You can make it last less or longer, depending on your commitments and the energy you want to dedicate to it. I advise you to stay at least 15 minutes as it is the time that I save and find most useful.

For the location, I advise you to sit down, avoiding lying down. Because you could relax too much and fall asleep, at your discretion, you can prefer a chair rather than a comfortable pillow to stay on the ground.

The important thing is that you have to feel comfortable because you will have to maintain the exercise duration.

Keep your back straight. Take on the correct posture, straightening your back and pulling your head up. Imagine you have a thread over your back, and someone pulls it up.

Make sure you don't stiffen your muscles, back, or shoulders too much. Relax your body.

Breathe!

Take some deep breaths to relax the body and mind. Focus only on the air that enters from the nose and drops to the stomach, and then goes up and out of the mouth.

Meditation

Learn to connect with the silence within yourself and understand that everything in this life has a purpose.

If you already have a meditative experience, you will surely have noticed how, with simple breathing, you are already meditating.

To increase your ability to concentrate, a meditative exercise consists precisely of focusing only on your breath. For self-hypnosis, I recommend using this experience of yours as a basis. Let us now add a few details.

Find Peace

Keep focusing on your breath. Watch your thoughts flow before you. The aim is not to be influenced by them. Imagine yourself on the bank of a stream as you watch the water flow in front of you.

Your thoughts are like flowing water, so they'll pass you by, but just as quickly, they'll leave. If ideas come in that lead you to a negative emotional state, drive them away. Do not fight them, accept them, and let them flow.

Refrain from any form of judgment. Focus on peace and serenity. Cultivate these emotions within you until you hear them grow until they completely envelop you.

To achieve this state, you can mentally repeat a mantra that will help you stay focused on your goal.

"I'm calm, and I'm at peace."

Enjoy

Allow yourself to stay as much as you wish, wrapped in this pleasant and comfortable feeling of calm and serenity.

Stay in your paradise, and enjoy the present. Pay attention and think carefully about what you're feeling. Give yourself as much time as you need. You can help by associating what you think with a word, for example: "PEACE." In this way, when you think of the word "peace," it will be easier for you to recall this feeling from your memory.

If your goal was to combat anxiety or stress, you might already decide to stop this meditative session. Otherwise, you are in the ideal condition to operate directly on your subconscious, to unleash your superpower!

The View

It is not enough to look. You have to look with eyes that want to see, that believe in what they see.

By the term visualization, I do not mean the ability to "see mentally," therefore, imagination, or rather, not only that! I am referring precisely to a total empathy of what you imagine by this word; seeing in detail what you want, taking advantage of all your five senses.

Observe every detail, shape, and color. Taste its taste. Tap with your hand to feel the sensation on your skin. Smell it and the sound it makes. Create a vivid mental scene full of all these details!

Identify the Goal

What's your purpose? What do you want to get from this exercise? For example, do you want to quit smoking, lose weight, exercise, find a soul mate, fight shyness, or increase your self-esteem? Choose a specific goal to develop and focus on the duration of the session.

You can ask for everything you want, and there are no limits!

Get It

Once you know what you want to achieve, focus all your energy on getting it. What do I mean? View, as I've shown you before, that you've already got what you want. Recreate in detail the scene you want to live and experience it! Allow yourself to feel pride and happiness for reaching your goal and making your dreams come true! You deserve it!

Stay Focused

Stay focused on your feelings, what you feel, and firmly believe you've already gotten it.

Turn away distractions, and don't let doubt creep into your thoughts! When you notice that this is happening, simply mentally relive your success and shift your attention to this emotion. Feel within you grow the power to shape your reality only with your will!

If you believe you have already gained it, then your trust in you, god, or the universe will only increase more and more!

Now you can come back. At this point, you are ready to interrupt the session and return to your daily activities.

Fix the emotions indelibly you feel, and feel free to recall and relive them whenever you want throughout the day!

Gradually return to reality, counting up to 5:

Repeat to yourself, "I am calm, and I am at peace."

Repeat to yourself, "I am sure of me and believe in my abilities."

Breathe. Shift your attention to the incoming air of your nose, go down and go up to get out of your mouth.

Shift your focus to your surroundings. Feel the sounds and smells around you.

Please open your eyes. "Thanks to my will, I will get what I desire."

Repetition

People keep on saying, "My life is miserable," and say they don't want to live in unhappiness, but they continue to shift the responsibility to something else, to someone else: fate, society, economic structure, the state, the church, the wife, the husband, the mother; anyway the manager is someone else.

The last ingredient of this magnificent self-hypnosis is its repetition. As I mentioned earlier, it takes time for these emotions and thoughts to take root and grow in our minds.

Try to carve out time daily to carry out this exercise. You will feel better and face the day with more energy charge!

Take advantage of the words you've associated with your moods to evoke when you want your mental images. Relive the scenes and hear them already yours. You can do this several times throughout the day, whenever you want!

Turn away negative thoughts and firmly believe in you and your success. This is the key, a secret that now belongs to you and that you can exploit to create your destiny!

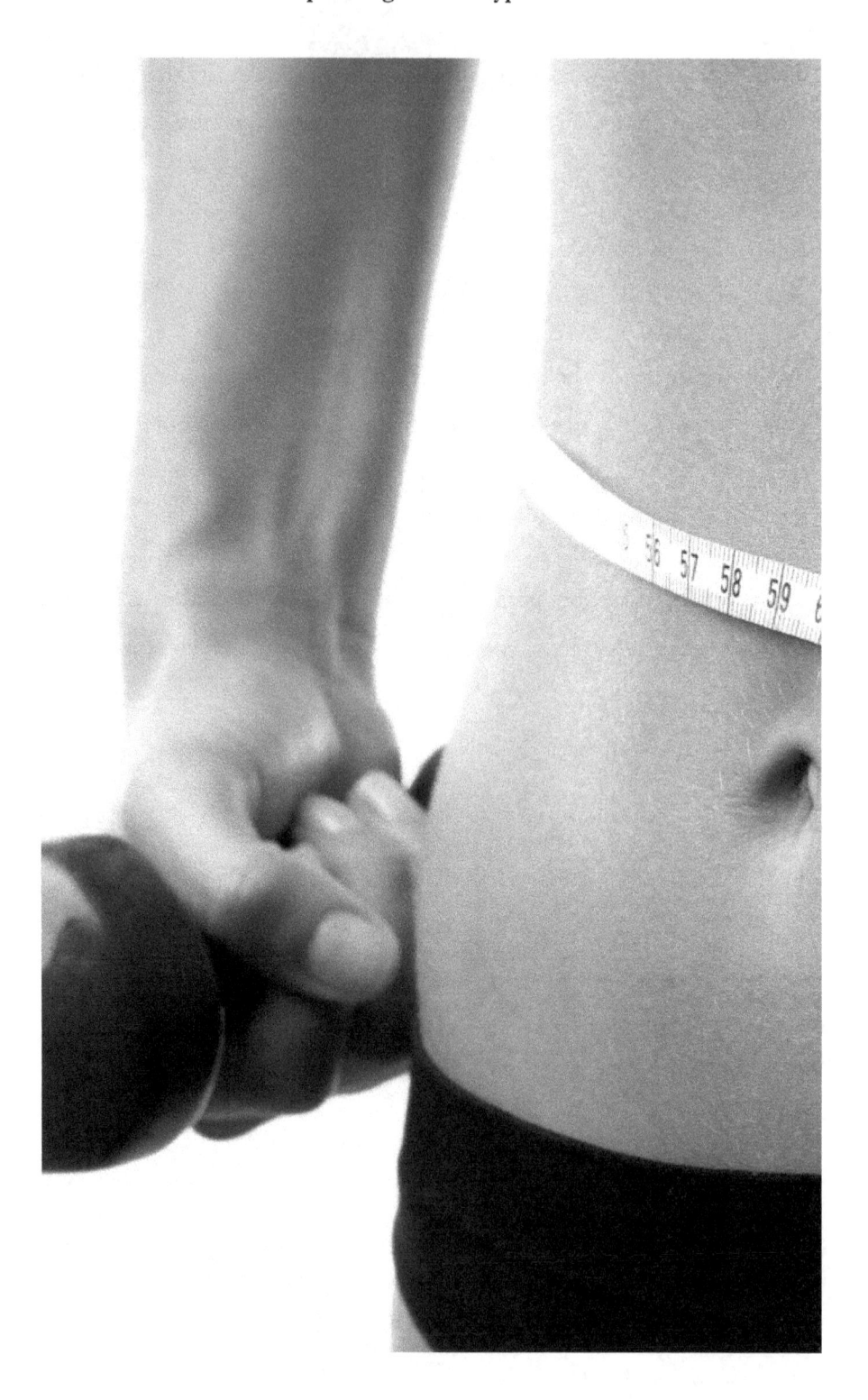

Chapter 10:
How to Hypnotize Yourself

After laying the necessary foundations to understand the process of how to hypnotize yourself, it's time to learn how to do a self-hypnosis session.

You're probably wondering now, "Does hypnosis work?" or "Can I hypnotize myself?"

To make it easy for you to reach a hypnosis state, I propose a gradual process, which will take you step by step from induction to visualization and finally to a gentle and regular exit from the hypnotic trance.

Before you start, it is essential to reflect on the right place to conduct the self-hypnosis session. If your environment is noisy or full of distractions, it is not the right place for this practice.

The ideal is to carry out the process in a quiet, comfortable, and reserved place where you will not be disturbed for as long as necessary. Many people like to lie on the bed during sessions, but you can also sit with a straight back and open shoulders.

When lying down, keep your feet resting on the mattress, with your knees slightly raised to form an angle of about 100 degrees. It's also worth considering the best time of day for self-hypnosis. For example, doing the session before bed allows you to fall asleep at the end of the process naturally, but you may also be too sleepy to focus on the viewing phase.

Alternatively, starting the morning with the hypnosis car can help you prepare for a positive and productive day.

It might be worth experimenting with both approaches to see what works best for you. Personally, the time when I practice hypnosis cars is about an hour after lunch. In this way, I use that time that many dedicate to a nib to rest and work on my unconscious, to be more energetic in the afternoon when the energies usually begin to wane.

Often some people create real hypnosis car walls, so I wrote an article in which I identify which are the six most frequent and show you how to overcome them.

Preparing for Self-Hypnosis

Preparing for hypnosis simply means getting into the right physical and mental state to get the most out of the session.

So, ask yourself: what helps me relax and unwind? There are no hard-and-fast rules that you have to follow. However, listening to relaxing music, doing yoga, taking a quiet walk in nature, or taking a bath with essential oils are excellent examples of ways you can slow down and concentrate your mind before hypnosis.

While finding the right environment and getting ready for the car are two essential steps to take before self-hypnosis, there are also other things worth doing before starting the session.

It is also essential to set an intention or motivation to turn into a verbal statement. In other words, you're going to benefit from knowing exactly why you're doing self-hypnosis.

Incorporate statements into your hypnosis. You may want to recite statements before starting each session, as well as at the end. These statements must be made positively.

For example, if you're trying to overcome anxiety about a sports presentation, avoid saying things like, "I don't have to play badly."

You prefer statements such as:

- Today I will give the best of myself

- I can access my full potential

- Play as concentrated and effective as possible

- Similarly, if you're looking to quit smoking, choose something like, "I feel healthy and happy without cigarettes."

Apart from using lively and stimulating language, there are no rules for what is right and wrong. As long as your words have a positive focus and make you feel good, you're on the right track.

Tuning

Doing a simple breathing exercise will help you get into the right state of mind for self-hypnosis. For example, you can spend 3 to 5 minutes breathing deeply, inhaling through the nose, and exhaling through the mouth.

When you do, help tune in the extraneous details by telling your mind and body that it's time for thoughtful, concentrated exercise. You may also benefit by exhaling longer than you breathe, which helps slow down your heart rate.

TIP: Imagine being in a train station and seeing a very long train pass by. There are so many thoughts, ideas, and distractions on every single carriage. Your job is to stay on the platform and let these thoughts keep passing. If you find yourself clinging to one of the carriages, you need to return to the forum. The more you practice hypnosis cars, the easier it will be to keep all your focus on exercise. Also, strengthening your concentration can benefit you for many other skills needed in everyday life.

Project Your Intentions

Focus all the power of your focus on the thing you want to change: the habit, feeling, or trait that blocks you. Think back to the intention you defined before you start hypnotizing yourself and repeat it to yourself with your chosen words.

He goes on to say, "I think I can change my habits/feelings/behaviors."

You can repeat these words aloud or in your head, depending on how you feel best.

Once you feel like you're completely immersed in your intention, and it's clear to you, project it outwards into the space around you.

Imagine it is a signal you're sending into the universe or as a commitment you're making for everyone to notice.

Breathe Deeply

This is the stage of self-hypnosis, in which you move beyond greater concentration and relaxation and begin to induce a trance.

First, go back to the breathing pattern you adopted initially, inhaling slowly and deeply through the nose and exhaling through the mouth. This time, you feel that you relax more and more with each breath, sinking further into a hypnotic state.

After several minutes, move your eyes upwards so that they look towards the top of the eyelids and towards the point where the third eye is said to be located (between the eyebrows).

Try to relax your eyes, and as you do so, notice the way your eyelids start beating.

There is no set time that you have to impose for this step; focusing on time will only distract you from the process.

Instead, take your time and allow yourself to dive. Again, this will probably become faster and easier with practice.

Implementation

At this point, you are in a relaxed state and are receptive to hypnotic suggestion. This means it's time to delve deeper into your trance before viewing your intention.

There are some practical ways to do this.

Beginners often say that they find it easy to view the stairs, which involves imagining yourself going down a flight of stairs. Many people often choose a spiral staircase.

Count as you descend the steps, from 10 to 0, and notice how your body becomes looser and more relaxed as you approach the bottom. When you reach the end of the stairs, you should feel calm, and your mind should be controlled.

An alternative way to deepen your trance is to imagine a scene that you find incredibly relaxing. For example, it could be a green lawn, a beautiful beach, or a quiet forest. It can be a place you've seen in real life, a scene from a movie, or an image you create in your imagination.

As with stairs, imagine your body getting more massive and more relaxed as you delve into the imagined scene. With both approaches, the goal is to slow down your thoughts, increase your receptiveness, and rise to a deep state of calm.

View

Visualization is a potent tool when used correctly and is critical to triggering a transformation in the trance state. This step triggers change and helps you change the behaviors, habits, or feelings that have held you back. First, imagine standing somewhere, perhaps in a quiet place (as described in the previous passage) or in a place where you have found meaningful memories.

Again, it can be real or imaginary. Then, reconnecting with your stated intention, start displaying yourself in line with those claims. What you want to do here is to imagine your best and most accomplished self.

So, for example, if you're trying to overcome the habit of procrastinating, imagine being highly productive and happy. So, get into that image, actually imagining yourself as the best self. To maximize this phase, we must allow our emotional responses to be generated much more readily than words alone.

Build this image with as many details as possible, including all your senses: sight, hearing, smell, and touch. Think about how you would feel, what you would do, and what you would attract in your life.

Emergence

When you feel that you have viewed yourself to your full potential and are immersed in the image you have created, you can work to get out of self-hypnosis.

The ideal is to plan ahead of your return from the hypnosis car. In particular, some people set an alarm clock on their smartphone (for example, with a peaceful piano melody or sounds of nature). Similarly, some people prefer a voluntary process, for example, by imagining going up the stairs that they have previously dropped, then counting from 1 to 10.

If you're using the image of the quiet place, instead, you might walk backwards until you can see the home only in the distance. This process can take time, patience, and discipline before you start experiencing any changes. If you are interested in speeding up the process, you can use hypnosis wizard audio programs.

The 3 Stages of Self-Hypnosis

When you're mesmerized, you enter a deeply relaxed and highly receptive state, where positive suggestions can overcome the barriers and defenses that your mind usually puts in place.

Contrary to popular belief, you're not sleeping during autohypnosis, so you'll still be able to choose to get out of the hypnotic trance whenever you wish—this means that self-hypnosis is safe to do on your own and that you'll still be able to pay attention immediately if something sudden requires your concentration.

But what's interesting is that the hypnosis car helps you change the way you think and act. Now that you have a basic idea of what hypnosis implies, we can move on to exploring the three stages of hypnosis car.

When they think about the hypnosis car, people usually imagine that it takes a long time to learn the techniques. As you'll see, each of the hypnosis stages uses skills that you may have already started developing elsewhere.

Step 1: Hypnotic Induction

In the induction phase, you begin to relax and free your mind.

This is very similar to what happens when you relax to fall asleep at night, as it requires slowing down thoughts, letting go of physical tension, and putting aside practical worries for another time.

Some people find the induction phase of self-hypnosis easy, while others may have difficulties (especially if they are very stressed).

Below I will describe some techniques to facilitate induction. After passing this stage the first few times, your body will begin to relax more quickly.

Step 2: Creative Visualization

Next, you enter the creative visualization phase of self-hypnosis, in which you begin to eradicate old useless beliefs and replace them with new and more productive ways of thinking.

This phase requires the use of imagination, a high level of concentration, and a constant commitment to bringing about the change you're working on.

In other words, your intentions must be aligned with what you are imagining if you want to succeed in creating positive change.

This is why hypnosis requires pre-planning and careful examination of your goals. It is also wise to set one goal at a time, processing them in order.

Step 3: Exiting Hypnotic State

When you're done with the central part of self-hypnosis, it's time to get out of the hypnotic state. This is easy, and you will return to full and everyday awareness.

At first, you may feel a bit sleepy, but you can go on naturally.

However, it can be jarring to get out of self-hypnosis abruptly, so many people find it useful to have a cue indicating that the session is over.

This can be a specific word, a counting process (for example, 1 to 10), or a slight music alarm. We will see the sample signals in more detail later in this guide.

The Effects of Auto Hypnosis on the Chemistry of the Organism

There are several things to understand, which serves to make you know the true scope of this technique. Often people attribute the ability to act on thoughts to the hypnosis car, which is true, but it is too reductive a statement. These states produce particular effects on the organism, increasing the production of certain chemicals:

- Serotonin

- Melatonin

- Endorphins

- Dhea

- Cortisol

- Gaba

Let's see in detail what they are and how they are useful to us.

Serotonin

There seems to be agreement on serotonin: is it a hormone or a neurotransmitter?

However, most researchers think it is a neurotransmitter found mainly in the brain, bowels, and blood platelets. It is a chemical responsible for mood regulation. Studies show that serotonin affects appetite, sleep, social behavior, memory, and sexual desire.

But, what exactly does it do?

As a neurotransmitter, serotonin allows nerve cells in the brain to communicate with each other. It also contributes to some critical bodily functions:

- Regulates bowels and appetite.

- Helps form clots when there is a wound.

- Encourage nausea and vomiting to expel toxic or harmful substances.

- It has a significant impact on mood and happiness levels.

- People with low serotonin levels can feel depressed and suffer from poor memory.

- As a result, by increasing serotonin levels, you should be able to increase your happiness levels.

Melatonin

Melatonin is a hormone produced in the pineal gland in the brain. It is responsible for regulating circadian rhythms, making possible the unconscious mechanism that makes us sleep at night and stay awake during the day.

This is the natural rhythm of the human body, and the pineal gland works to maintain that rhythm, suppressing melatonin by day and releasing it at night.

Like serotonin, melatonin is involved in many other bodily functions:

- It's an antioxidant.

- Has anti-inflammatory properties.

- Strengthens the immune system (although it is not yet clear how it faces).

- Fights cancer, Alzheimer's disease, and tinnitus.

Although the body produces melatonin, there are times when supply does not meet demand. For example, if you don't get enough sleep, or during disease, or in case you lead a stressful lifestyle.

Precisely in these cases, melatonin can be prescribed in the form of a pill specifically to treat sleep disorders. I guess you know perfectly well how important sleep is to the body: it helps to regenerate, invigorate and reenergize every system.

It gives the brain time to absorb and organize all the information with which it came into contact. Without the right amount of sleep, people become irritable.

Endorphins

Endorphins are neurotransmitters produced in the hypothalamus and pituitary glands. Their task is to relieve stress and pain. People with low levels of endorphins can suffer from depression, so the opposite is also true. The more endorphins are released, the happier you feel.

Dehydroepiandrosterone

A hormone in your body is known as the mother of all hormones and as a source of juvenile hormone. It is called dehydroepiandrosterone, which is abbreviated to DHEA for apparent reasons. DHEA is a steroid hormone produced by the adrenal glands, gonads, and brains. Its primary function is to synthesize estrogen and androgens.

For this reason, DHEA is designed to improve athletic performance, so any athlete who takes it as a supplement risks being banned by the World Anti-Doping Agency. Although DHEA is thought to have anti-aging properties, there is no evidence to support this claim. We know that the less DHEA you have, the fewer years of life you have left.

Other things we know about this are that:

- Makes the immune system more efficient.

- Balances the body's relationship between lean muscles and fat tissue.

- Helps maintain optimal brain function.

- People suffering from depression have less DHEA in their blood.

Cortisol

When stress occurs, the body produces cortisol. Cortisol is the stress hormone produced in the adrenal glands located in the upper part of the kidneys.

It is best known for the role in the response of struggle or flight, giving the energy and strength necessary to deal with a crisis. Cortisol receptors are found in almost all cells in the body. This is because cortisol plays a role in several different functions, including:

- The regulation of blood pressure.

- Managing blood sugar levels.

- Controlling how the body uses carbohydrates, proteins, and fats.

- Contributes to circadian rhythm (sleep-wake cycle).

- Despite its bad reputation, stress is not as bad as it sounds.

If you didn't feel stressed, you wouldn't be able to react to dangers or threats. In these types of situations, your body emits extra cortisol to help you cope with everything.

Your heart rate accelerates, and more blood flows to the main muscle groups. Once the threat is addressed or the danger has passed, the systems should return to normal.

If they don't, there's too much cortisol, so too much stress; that's when it becomes a problem!

Similarly, if a person has a lifestyle that continually puts him or her under stress, he or she may produce more cortisol than necessary.

This means that his body never has a chance to calm down and can lead to some health problems, such as:

- Headache.

- Diseases of the heart.

- Digestion problems.

- Difficulty sleeping.

- Memory and concentration issues.

Anxiety and Depression

It is not a secret that hypnosis is one of the best natural stress techniques.

Even a simple necessary hypnotic induction helps to focus on breathing and the search for deep relaxation. Of course, the more relaxed you are, the less stressed you are.

This is important because the body automatically adjusts the amount of cortisol produced as needed.

When you are happily relaxed in a peaceful hypnotic trance, there is no need for further cortisol production. So you have the power to turn it off and enjoy some time in serenity and stress-free, using nothing but simple necessary induction.

Gamma-Aminobutyric Acid

According to the World Health Organization, mental illness accounts for about 15% of the world's diseases, with depression and anxiety disorders leading the way.

Both depression and anxiety are also associated with low levels of GABA (gamma-aminobutyric acid).

GABA is a neurotransmitter that has the task of slowing down or inhibiting nerve cells in the brain. In this way, it helps control fear and anxiety, which is why GABA is sometimes also called a calming chemical.

Interestingly, researchers from Boston University School of Medicine (BUSM) and McLean Hospital found that trance status could increase a person's GABA levels.

But why should a person increase their GABA levels?

Therefore, low levels of GABA are believed to contribute to anxiety and depression. Similarly, it is thought that rising levels can improve mood and stimulate the nervous system's relaxation.

People take GABA as a supplement in an attempt to:

- Improving mood.

- Eliminating anxiety.

- Sleep better.

Dealing with Premenstrual Syndrome

But, wouldn't it be better to increase your GABA levels naturally?

Without having to fill your body with supplements that may or may not produce the required effect. All this is what is stimulated when you are within the trance state. That's why I always recommend a good practice of hypnosis cars.

How long does the proper practice of hypnosis cars last? These are the benefits of hypnosis from a strictly chemical perspective.

If we add the element of suggestions, what happens is that in addition to being released these substances, you can guide the unconscious to make essential changes and evoke resources useful to achieve their goals. Of course, it is essential to specify that this is a practice and not a magic wand.

Many people believe that they will achieve incredible results after using a hypnosis technique (and maybe all the chemical elements mentioned will stabilize forever). Unfortunately, if they think this is not necessarily their fault, the publicity made by people who have made science promises.

Believing such lies is like believing that it will take a day in the gym to have the body you want or that you just have to fast for a few days to get back to your shape weight and never pick up an ounce again.

I'm sorry, but it doesn't work that way. Being a practice, it is a work on oneself that needs patience.

How much patience in terms of time?

Let's see it now!

The ideal is to practice hypnosis for about 30 minutes a day. This is the time it takes for the body to release the chemicals we saw above. To start seeing the first benefits, you need to wait about fifteen days. This does not mean that you do not feel better after the hypnosis car session, but to see something more important than simple relief, you need to wait a while.

After about three months of practice, the callous body begins to thin, the layer that divides the two hemispheres of our brain: this produces a more remarkable ability to think, reflect, act and, consequently, achieve the results we want.

The mistake that people who practice hypnosis car make (and I repeat, we've seen who's to blame) is not to give us proper weight and attention.

Taking care of one's mind should be a daily activity, as we do when we take care of our body: every day, we wash, feed, and the most attentive practice sports.

In this way, we manage to make our body as functional as possible, allowing it to offer us the best and preserve it for as long as possible. With the hypnosis car, we do precisely the same thing but with our minds.

This is why more and more successful athletes, artists, and managers are using it: it improves both physical and mental performance.

Small But Essential Additional Tips

In this section, I want to discuss some finesse that can help you manage your hypnosis car in the best way.

Up to this point, we have seen how to practice it and its benefits.

Now, I want to show you some subtleties that you can integrate to overcome any snags you might find and carry yourself with the hypnosis car in the most precise and functional way possible.

What to Do if I Don't Relax?

I've already told you how breathing can be useful in these cases. What I want to show you now is a somewhat more complex breathing technique, which is divided into three phases:

- **Step 1:** Inhale from the nose, counting four times.

- **Step 2:** Three-stroke holdings.

- **Step 3:** Exhale from the mouth, counting five times.

This form of breathing should be practiced for about five minutes.

In case you are not yet relaxed enough, you can follow a contraction and relaxation strategy. This consists of contracting all the muscles in your body for about ten seconds and then letting them go.

Do this about three times. In this way, your muscles will tend to relax spontaneously as a result of previous contractions. These two sequential strategies can be beneficial in preparing both the mind and the body for hypnosis.

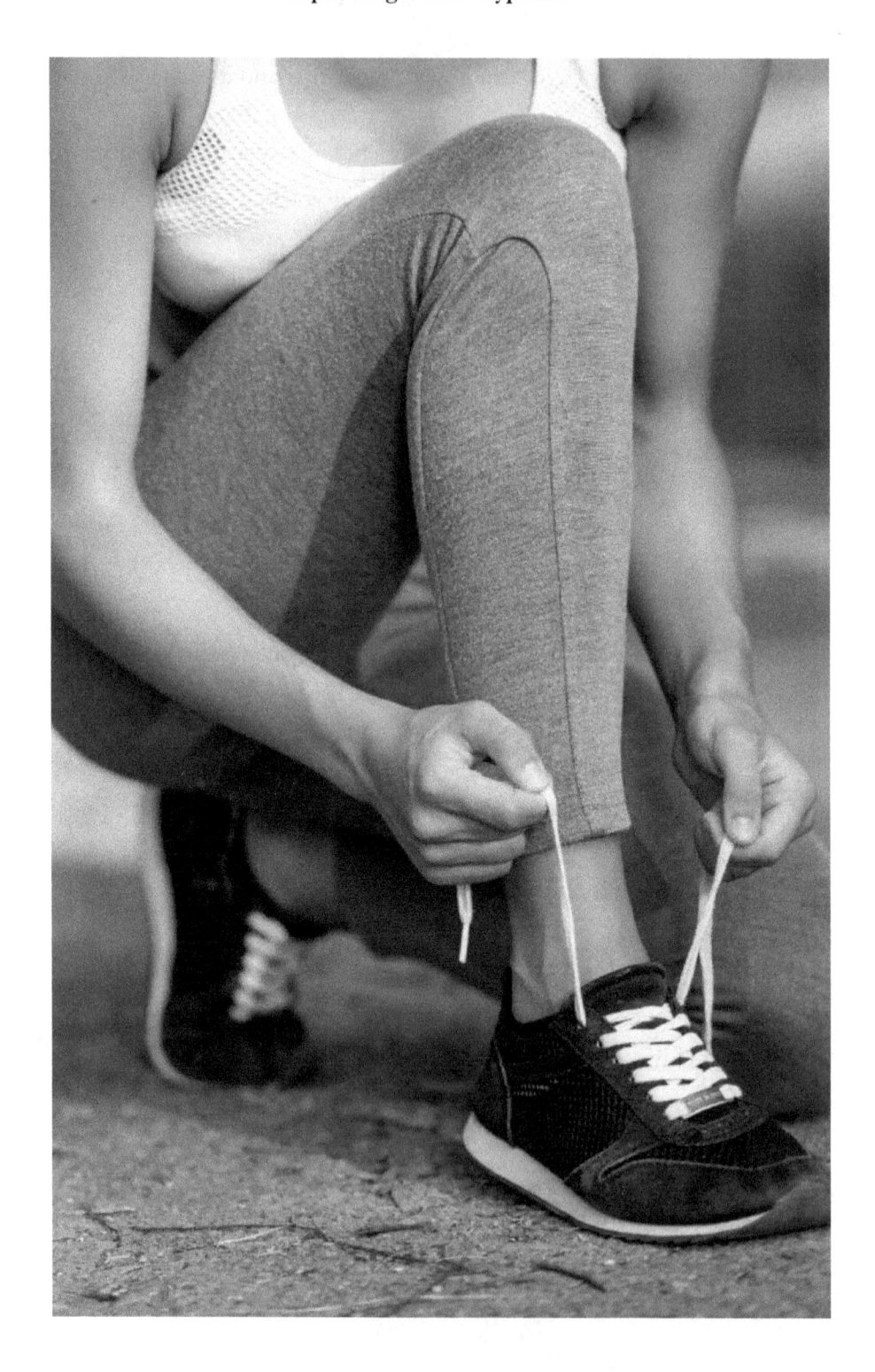

Conclusion

The unconscious believes that a Gastric Band has been installed through hypnosis and causes the stomach to respond as if it had it physically installed (virtual stomach reduction), causing patients to eat less because they believe that their stomach has reduced its size and capacity, feeling satiated much earlier.

That way, they manage to lose weight until they reach their ideal weight. It's not about dieting or banning anything (the prohibition engenders even more desire about what is prohibited).

The application of hypnotic techniques, specific suggestions, and mental reprogramming to achieve a healthier, more appropriate eating habit definitively free yourself from food anxiety.

It is guiding and designed for both professional hypnotherapists and psychologists with hypnosis training; they must be trained in Therapeutic Hypnosis or possess a Degree in Psychology.

In both cases, students gain the necessary knowledge to apply the Virtual Gastric Band professionally (under hypnosis).

CPSIA information can be obtained
at www.ICGtesting.com
Printed in the USA
LVHW051147100621
689814LV00002B/80